# PREFACE

This picture quiz atlas aims to be of interest and help to those training in otolaryngology. Ear, nose and throat ailments are however common, and those in general practice, or in specialities that overlap with otolaryngology, as well as medical students, may enjoy perusing the pictures and text, testing their powers of observation and ability to make diagnoses. This atlas is intended as 'light' reading, and I hope information of practical use, for those dealing with otolaryngological problems, will be acquired.

# ACKNOWLEDGEMENTS

I would like to thank David Jonathan, Senior Registrar at The Royal National Throat Nose and Ear Hospital, for testing himself on these quiz questions, and advising on their clarity and fairness.

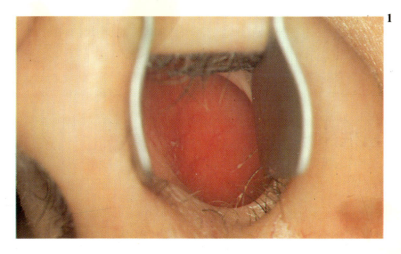

1 (a) What area of the nose is being examined?
(b) Why is this area significant?
(c) Which blood vessels supply this area?


2 This patient presented with irritation and discomfort over the right side of the face and nose with nasal obstruction.
(a) What nerve supplies this area of skin?
(b) What is the probable diagnosis?

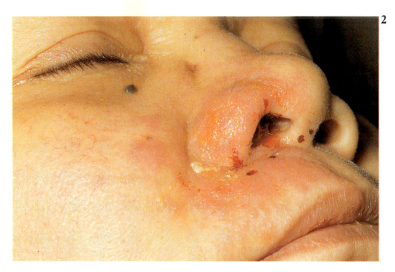

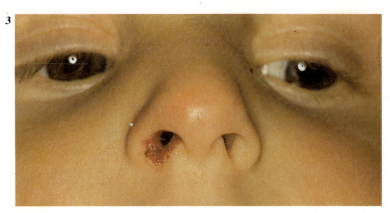

**3** This five-year-old child presented with a three-week history of soreness and irritation of the right nostril associated with an unpleasant discharge.
(a) What is the diagnosis?
(b) What is a possible differential diagnosis?


**4** This seven-year-old child complained of right nasal obstruction following nasal injury.
(a) What is the diagnosis?
(b) In what simple way may this be confirmed?

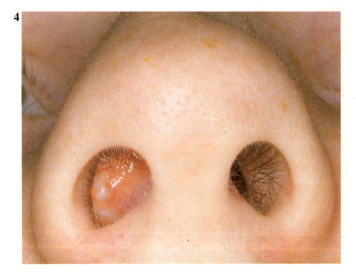

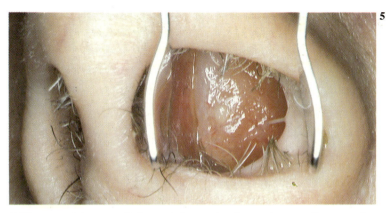

**5** The complaint was of left nasal obstruction increasing over four months, with occasional epistaxis.
(a) What does examination of the left nares show?
(b) What are the possible diagnoses?

**6** On performing the Valsalva manoeuvre the right side of this patient's neck expanded.
(a) What is the probable diagnosis?
(b) How may this relate to occupation?

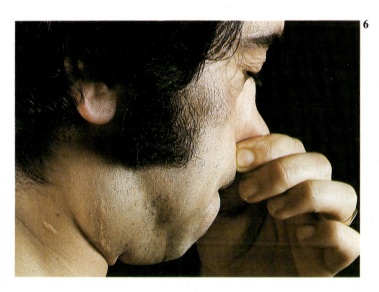

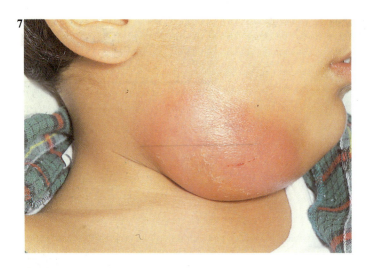

**7** This ten-year-old boy presented with this fluctuant mass, after a five-day period of painful swelling over the right cheek. Give two probable diagnoses.

**8** This inflammatory neck swelling settled rapidly with antibiotics but recurred. Once the acute infection had settled, there was little to see or feel in the neck.
(a) What is the diagnosis?
(b) What points are to be noted carefully on examination?

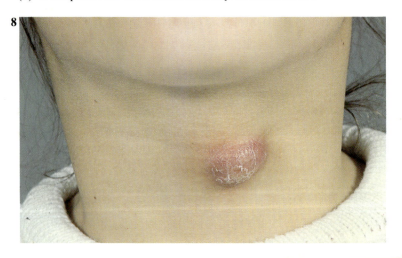

**9** (a) What is apparent in this lateral x-ray of the nasal bones?
(b) What nasal deformity usually necessitates this procedure?
(c) What is the possible long-term problem?

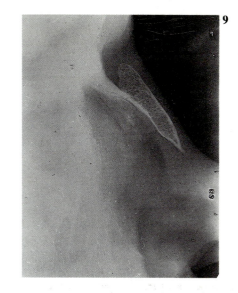

**10** (a) What nasal structure is demonstrated in this operative photograph?
(b) What operation is being carried out?

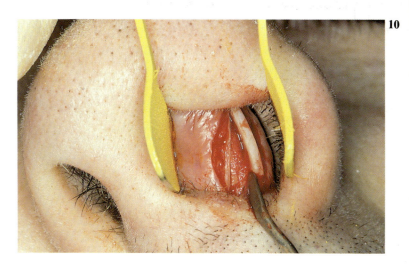

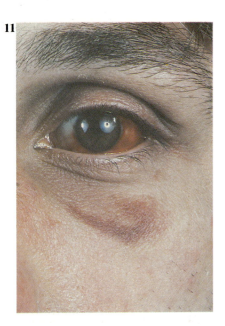

**11** Two days after a punch on the nose, this man complained that his eyelids closed when he blew his nose. He was concerned with the appearance of the eye.

(a) What condition has caused the intermittent eye swelling?

(b) What injuries associated with a nasal fracture should be excluded?

**12** This diagram shows a coronal section through the larynx indicating the ventricular band, vocal cord and subglottic regions.

(a) Which is the commonest site for a carcinoma of the larynx?

(b) Is the prognosis for this condition good?

(c) What is the treatment?

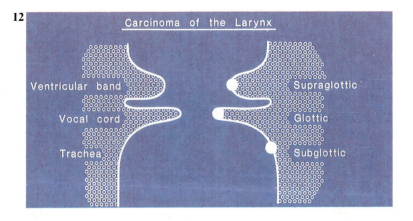

Carcinoma of the Larynx

Ventricular band

Vocal cord

Trachea

Supraglottic

Glottic

Subglottic

**13** This 12-year-old girl complained that she did not like the appearance of her nose.
(a) What syndrome is apparent?
(b) What operation would be needed to improve the appearance?

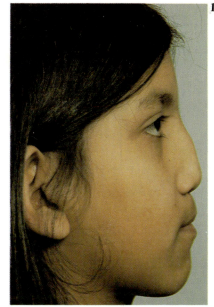

**14** Examination of this patient's nasal vestibule showed this white area.
(a) What is the diagnosis?
(b) How is this caused?
(c) What direct question should this patient be asked?

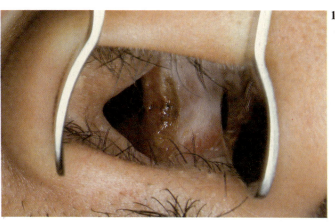

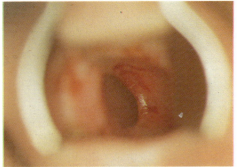

**15** This patient complained of intermittent epistaxis.
(a) What does examination reveal?
(b) What habit or occupation may be related to this finding?

**16** This adolescent complained of unilateral nasal obstruction. Examination of the oropharynx revealed a greyish swelling below the soft palate.
(a) What is the diagnosis?
(b) What steps can be made to confirm this?
(c) What does an antral proof puncture reveal?

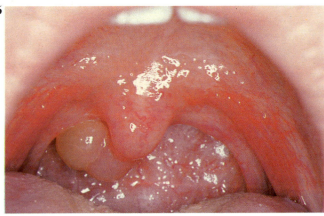

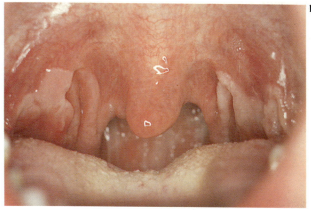

**17** Examination of a patient complaining of a sore throat revealed irregular superficial ulcers involving the tonsils and soft palate.
(a) Of which condition are the ulcers characteristic?
(b) What test should be carried out for confirmation?

**18** This patient's ear had lost its normal appearance and on palpation was soft. There had also been a collapse of the nasal dorsum and a complaint of hoarseness with tenderness over the larynx.
(a) What is the diagnosis?
(b) What further examination of the ear can confirm this?

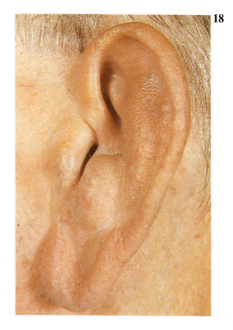

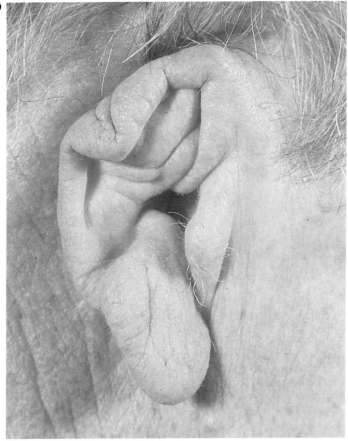

**19** This patient had lost the normal anatomy of the pinna which had 'collapsed'. This had been long-standing and dated from an infection 20 years earlier.
(a) What infection causes this appearance?
(b) What is the organism involved?

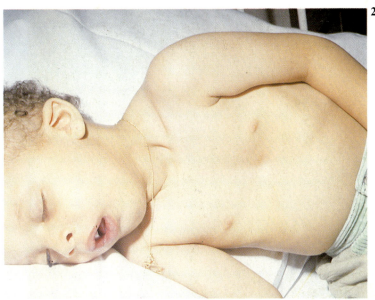

**20** This child, with marked nasal obstruction and mouth breathing during the daytime, is a prolific snorer. There is a complaint of hearing loss and episodes of sore throat.
(a) What is the probable cause of the snoring?
(b) What diagnosis must be excluded and further tests carried out?
(c) What is the cause of the hearing loss?
(d) What signs are obvious on examination of this child?

**21**

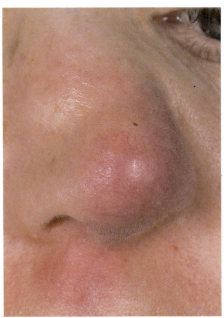

**21** This middle-aged woman complained of an increasing nasal deformity with 'saddling' of the nose. There was also nasal obstruction.
(a) What does this photograph show?
(b) What is the probable diagnosis?

**22** (a) What abnormality does examination of the anterior nares of this patient show?
(b) What structure gives rise to this?

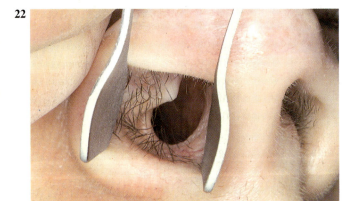

**22**

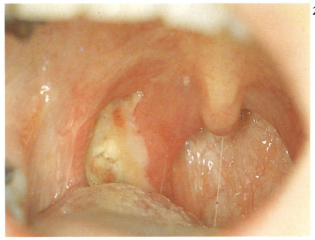

**23** Five days after a tonsillectomy, the patient was concerned to have noticed this yellow/white appearance of the fauces. What does this appearance represent?

**24** When protruded, the tongue deviated to the left and the surface was seen to fibrillate. There was a long-standing complaint of increasing left-sided hearing loss with pulsating tinnitus.
(a) What is the probable diagnosis?
(b) What cranial nerves are involved?

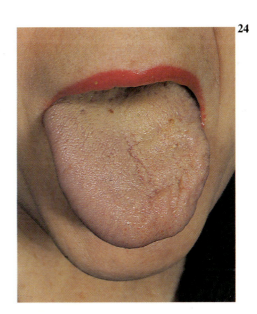

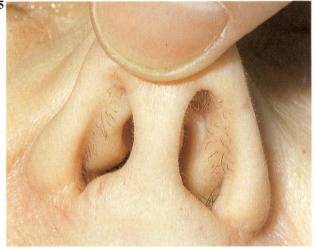

**25** What factors demonstrated on examination of this patient's nasal vestibule may contribute to the symptom of nasal obstruction?

**26** This middle-aged man had a swelling below the left ear, but also presented with this apparently large left tonsil.
(a) Is the tonsil enlarged?
(b) What is the probable diagnosis?

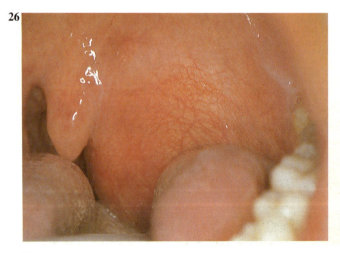

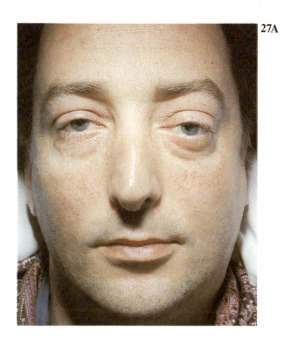

27 (a) What abnormality is apparent with this patient's left orbit?
(b) What nasal condition commonly causes this appearance?
(c) What may be relevant in the past history?

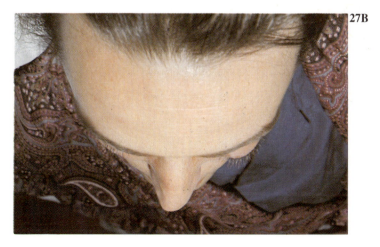

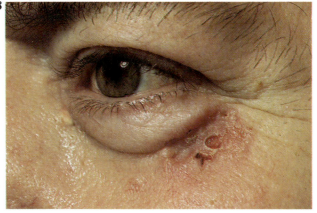

**28** This patient presented with a long-standing ulceration below his left eye.
(a) What is the diagnosis?
(b) What tests are carried out to confirm this?
(c) What is the treatment?

**29** An 18-year-old presented with malaise and sore throat.
(a) What are the characteristics of the fauces?
(b) What is the diagnosis?
(c) Is ampicillin the antibiotic of choice?

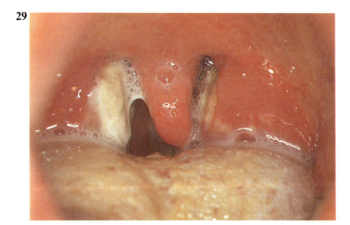

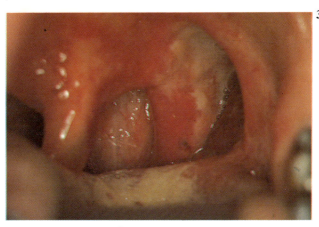

**30** Five days after tonsillectomy there was a complaint of increased throat pain and bleeding.
(a) What is seen on examination of these fauces?
(b) What is the diagnosis?
(c) What is the management?

**31** (a) Examination of the left anterior naris demonstrates what pathology?
(b) What cartilage and bone are involved in this abnormality?
(c) What operation is required to relieve the nasal obstruction?

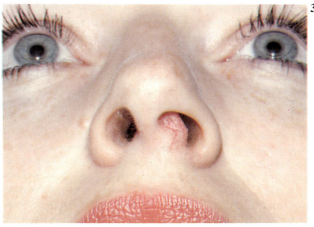

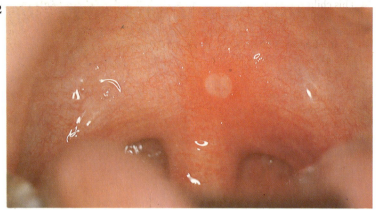

**32** This patient complained of a sore throat following a general anaesthetic.
(a) What lesion is apparent?
(b) What may have triggered this?
(c) What may be relevant in the past history?

**33** (a) What are these x-rays and what anatomical structure do they mainly show?
(b) What pathology is demonstrated in **B**?
(c) What is the probably diagnosis?

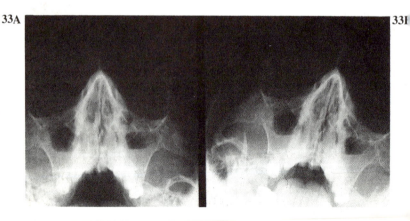

33A        33B

**34** This child was born with a pinna deformity affecting one ear only.
(a) Is treatment necessary for the associated conductive hearing loss on this side?
(b) Is pinna reconstruction a straightforward procedure and what are the alternatives?

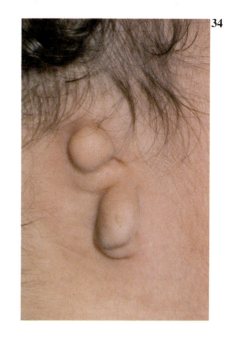

**34**

**35** This ten-year-old boy from Sicily presented with neck ulceration of four months' duration.
(a) Which structures in which site appear to be involved?
(b) What is the probable diagnosis?

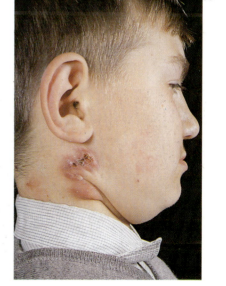

**35**

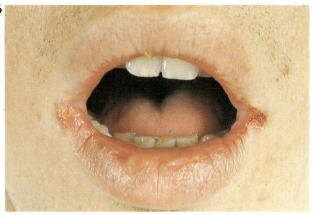

**36** (a) What is this condition affecting the angles of the mouth?
(b) What other symptoms and signs involving the throat may be associated with this?
(c) What is this syndrome and what is the possible long-term complication?

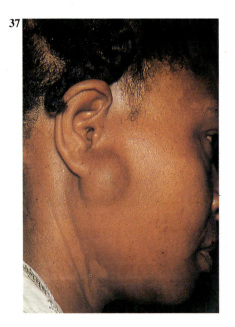

**37** This preauricular swelling of three months' duration is slightly tender on palpation.
(a) What is the diagnosis?
(b) What are the differential diagnoses?

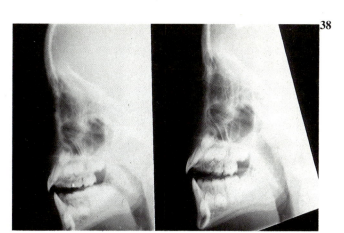

**38** Two x-rays of the same postnasal space are seen. In the one on the left there is occlusion of the postnasal space with enlarged adenoids. The postnasal space is relatively clear on the right side. What is the explanation?

**39** This patient's left palatal region pulsates and the tonsil is pushed to the mid-line. What is the probable diagnosis?

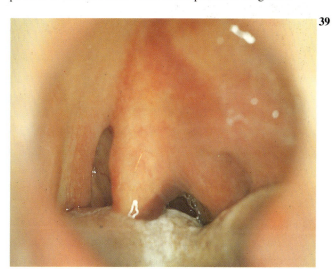

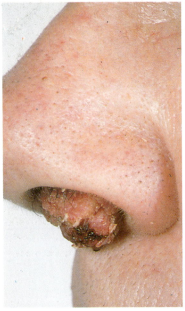
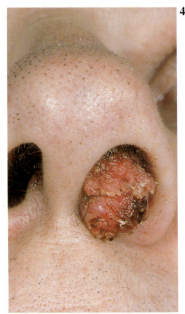

**40**  This middle-aged patient presented with this obvious nasal lesion and a long history of left epistaxis. There were no other symptoms or signs.
(a)  What are the possible diagnoses?
(b)  What are the characteristics that make the diagnosis of a simple nasal polyp unlikely?
(c)  What is the treatment?

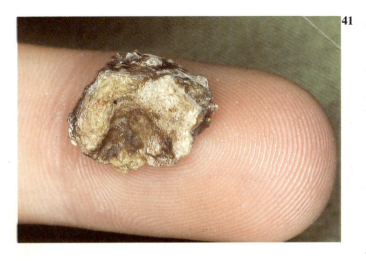

**41** This stoney, hard swelling was removed from the left nasal fossa.
(a) What is the diagnosis?
(b) What is the cause?
(c) Are there any complications?

**42** A complaint of irritation and tenderness over the ear lobe, with some tender cervical lymphadenopathy are the presenting signs. What is the probable cause?

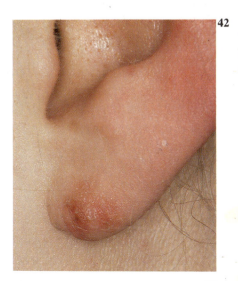

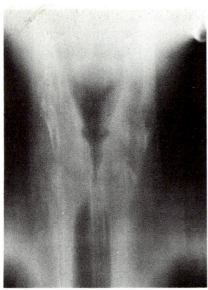

**43** (a) What type of x-ray is this?
(b) What pathology is apparent?

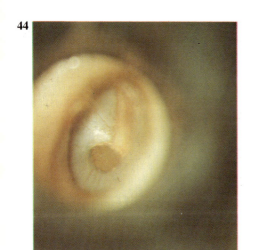

**44** A thin scar is apparent on this drum that, at first sight, appears to have an anterior perforation. What simple instrument is useful to be certain a perforation is not present?

**45** An elderly diabetic presented with a painful left ear with granulation tissue.
(a) What is the diagnosis?
(b) What will biopsy reveal?
(c) What organisms will be cultured from the discharge?

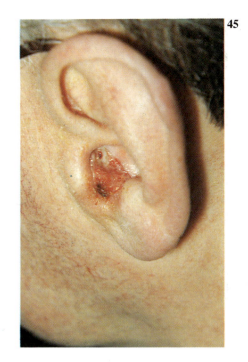

**46** (a) What investigation is being used for this patient?
(b) What abnormality is demonstrated?
(c) What may give rise to this appearance?
(d) In what instance may this technique still be of interest?

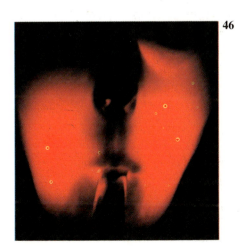

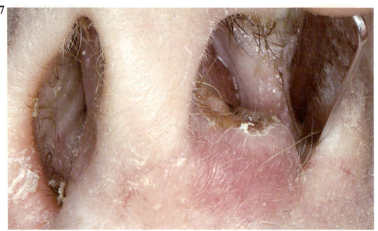

**47** This patient complained of a scanty blood-stained nasal discharge occurring over a period of six months.
(a) What does examination reveal?
(b) What are the steps in confirming diagnosis?
(c) What is the probable diagnosis?

**48** (a) What is this tonsillar excrescence which is symptom-free and firm on palpation with a probe?
(b) What is the treatment?

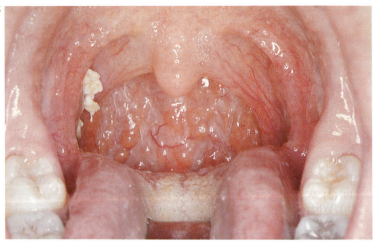

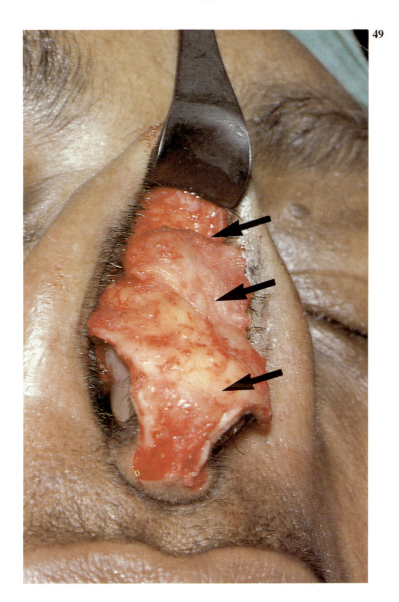

**49** (a) What nasal structures are arrowed?
(b) What operation is being carried out?

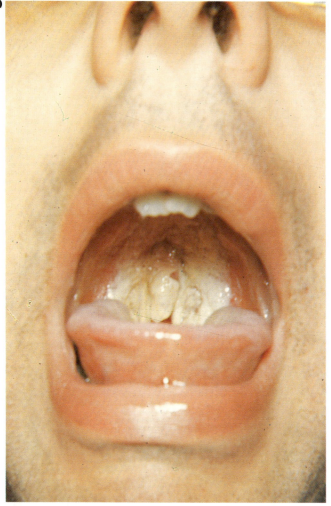

**50** A course of antibiotics did not improve this patient's symptoms of sore throat.
(a) What is the probable diagnosis?
(b) What will the throat swab reveal?
(c) What is the treatment?

**51** (a) What nerve distribution does this skin lesion involve?
(b) What is the diagnosis?

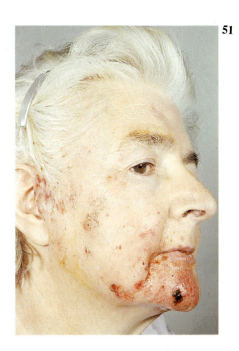

**52** What conditions may result in this severe palatal scarring?

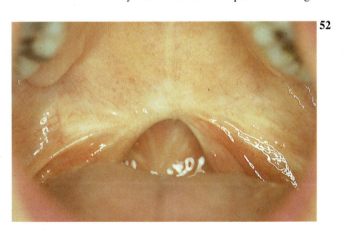

**53**

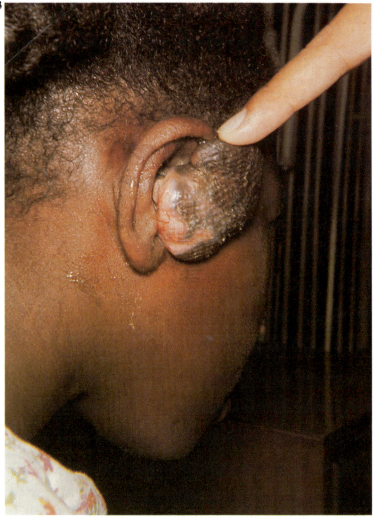

**53** There was a history of a previous operation in this 12-year-old girl who presented with a pedunculated preauricular swelling.
(a) What is the probable diagnosis?
(b) What lesion in this site may have required surgery?
(c) Is recurrence after further excision likely?

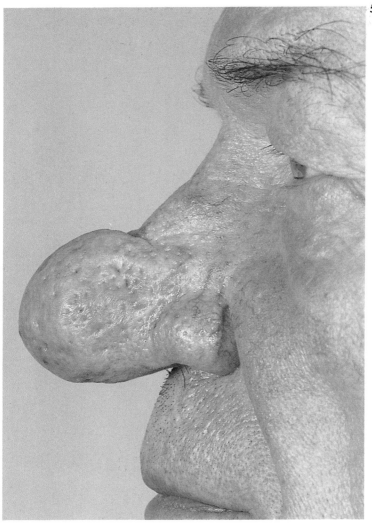

**54** (a) What is the diagnosis?
(b) What is the treatment?
(c) Is biopsy necessary?

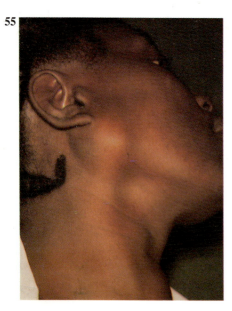

**55** (a) What is the site of this swelling?
(b) What is the probable diagnosis?
(c) What is the treatment?

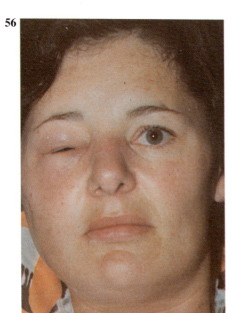

**56** A painful, tender swelling over the right cheek had persisted for ten days. There was no dental or maxillary sinus problem. What is the likely diagnosis?

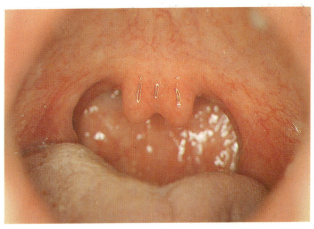

**57** (a) What abnormality is apparent in this oropharynx?
(b) With what symptoms is this associated?
(c) With what other physical signs may this abnormality be associated?

**58** (a) What is the abnormality apparent on examination of this oropharynx?
(b) What are the possible diagnoses?
(c) What management is usually necessary?

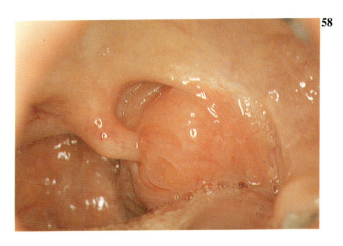

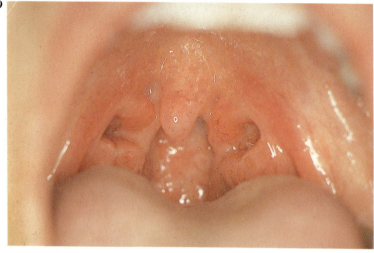

**59** (a) What are the abnormalities apparent in this patient's tonsils?
(b) With what symptoms may these be associated?
(c) What treatment may be necessary?

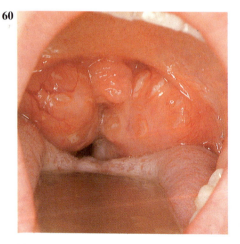

**60** These tonsils meet in the mid-line. What factors may be relevant to this finding?

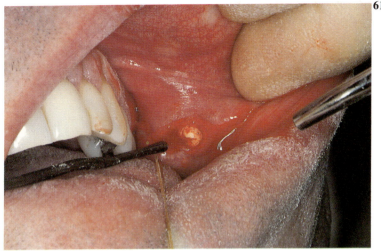

**61** This patient complained of painful swelling over the left cheek.
(a) What is the diagnosis?
(b) What treatment is being carried out?
(c) Is this condition common?

**62** (a) What abnormality is demonstrated?
(b) Is this usually associated with a speech defect?
(c) What treatment is required?

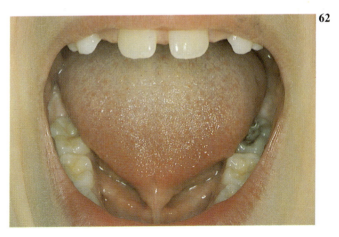

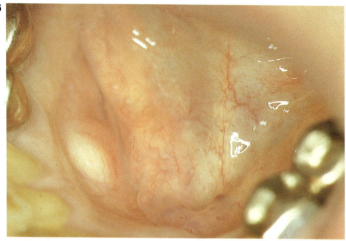

**63** (a)This white, bony, hard swelling in the floor of the mouth and on the inner aspect of the mandible, is characteristic of which lesion? (b) What treatment is required?

**64** (a) What is the diagnosis?
(b) What investigations are necessary?
(c) What is the treatment?
(d) What is a possible differential diagnosis?

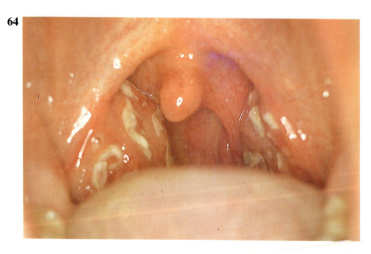

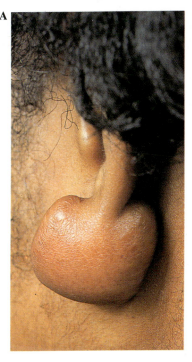 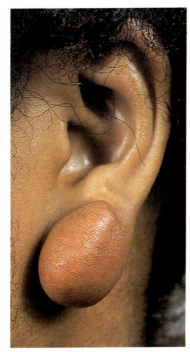

**65** (a) What is the probable diagnosis accounting for this firm, non-tender swelling of the ear lobule?
(b) What is the differential diagnosis?
(c) Is the treatment of this lesion straightforward?

**66** (a) What is the spot diagnosis of this lesion?
(b) What tests are necessary to confirm the diagnosis?

**67** (a) On what part of the pinna is this lesion?
(b) What are the possible diagnoses?
(c) What is the probable management required?

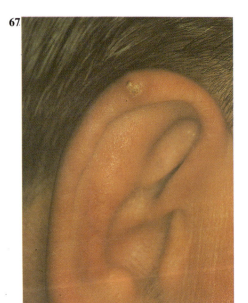

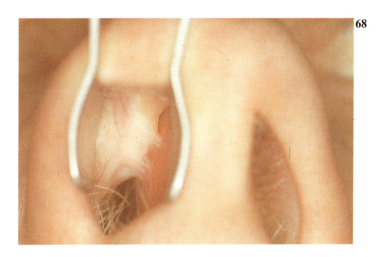

**68** (a) What abnormality does examination of this nasal vestibule show?
(b) What is the probable cause?
(c) What is the management?

**69** This patient complained of nasal obstruction which was more marked on the right side.
(a) What is the diagnosis?
(b) What treatment is required?

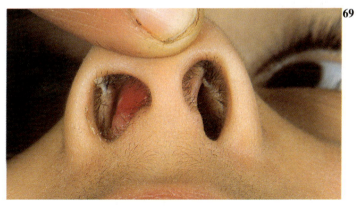

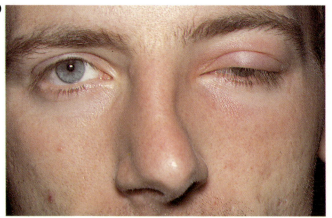

**70** This young man, with an external deviation of the nose and septal deviation to the left, developed pain and eye swelling with severe frontal headache, following a head cold.
(a) What is the probable diagnosis?
(b) What investigations are necessary to confirm this?
(c) What treatment is necessary?
(d) Are any complications probable, which should be watched for and excluded?

**71** There is a lesion in the floor of the left nasal vestibule.
(a) What is the probable diagnosis?
(b) What treatment is required?

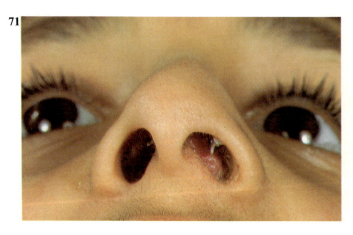

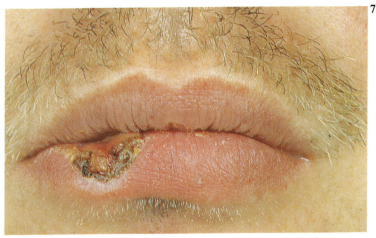

**72** Following minor trauma to the lip, this ulcer developed.
(a) What is the probable diagnosis?
(b) What investigations are necessary?


**73** (a) What does examination of this oropharynx demonstrate?
(b) What are the possible diagnoses?

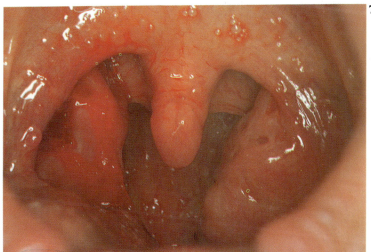

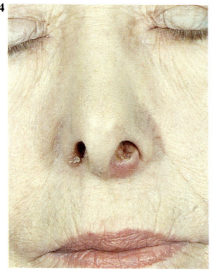

**74** This elderly woman presented with a painful ulcer in the left nasal vestibule, which had been increasing in size over the previous three months.
(a) What is the possible diagnosis?
(b) How can this be confirmed?

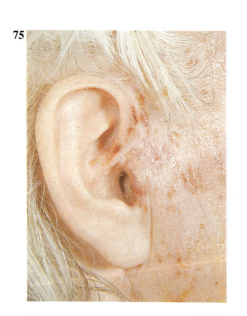

**75** A painful right ear with a sensorineural hearing loss developed suddenly with an associated preauricular skin eruption.
(a) What is the possible diagnosis?
(b) What other findings are probable?

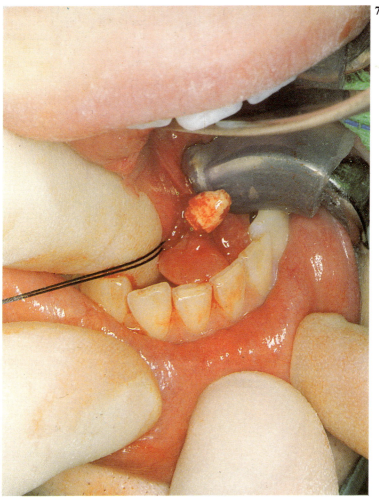

**76** This patient complained of swelling in the submandibular triangle on eating and drinking.
(a) What is the diagnosis?
(b) What procedure is being carried out?
(c) Is this always curative?

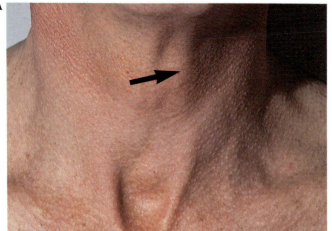

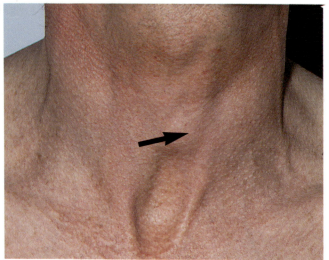

**77** (a) What characteristics do these photographs demonstrate of this neck swelling?
(b) What is the diagnosis?
(c) What treatment is usually required?
(d) What structure in continuity with the cyst requires excision to avoid recurrence.

**78** (a) What lesion is demonstrated in this tympanic membrane?
(b) What are the possible causes?
(c) What is the treatment?
(d) What is the prognosis?

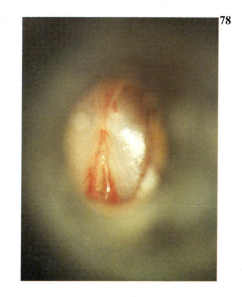

**79** (a) What investigation is being carried out?
(b) Name two conditions in which this investigation is particularly helpful in diagnosis?
(c) In what aural conditions is this investigation contraindicated?

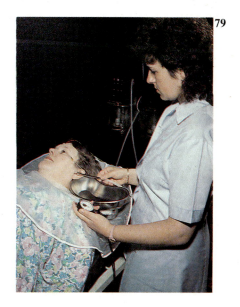

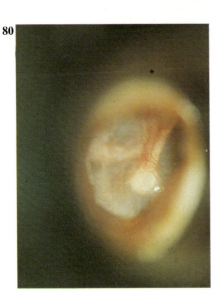

**80** Examination of this right tympanic membrane with the auroscope shows a line traversing the postero-superior segment of the tympanic membrane.
(a) What is this structure?
(b) What is its significance?

**81** (a) What abnormality does this fibreoptic photograph of the tympanic membrane show?
(b) What is the underlying pathology?
(c) What treatment may be necessary?

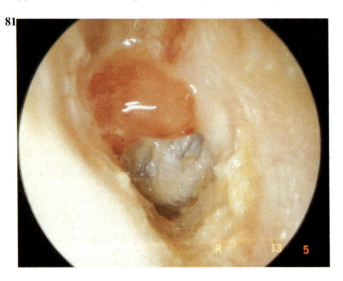

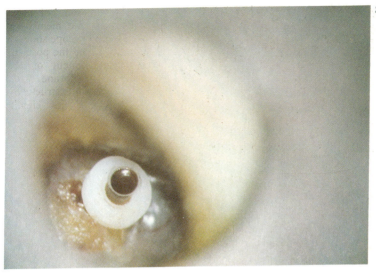

**82** (a) What does this photograph demonstrate?
(b) For what condition is this procedure carried out?
(c) What complication is apparent?

**83** (a) What does this tympanic membrane photograph demonstrate?
(b) Is this lesion 'safe'?
(c) What symptoms may result from this particular lesion?
(d) What treatment may be necessary?

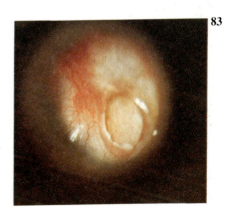

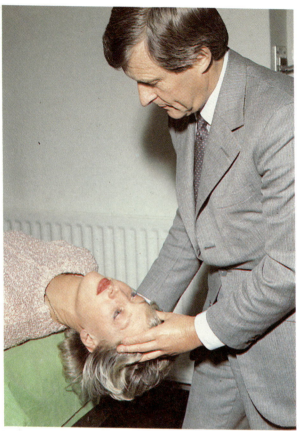

**84** (a) What clinical investigation is being carried out?
(b) For which particular condition is the test diagnostic?

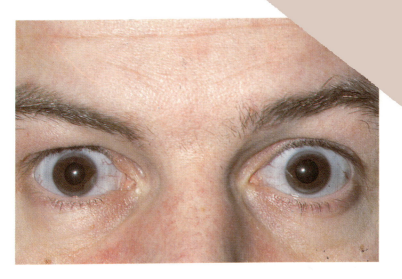

**85** (a) What abnormality of colour do this patient's sclerae show?
(b) With what aural condition are they associated?
(c) With what other condition may these particular sclerae be found?

**86** (a) What abnormality is seen in this left tympanic membrane?
(b) Name three structures that are apparent in the middle ear.

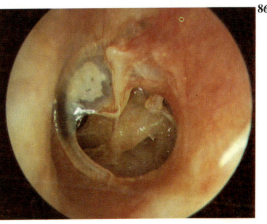

86

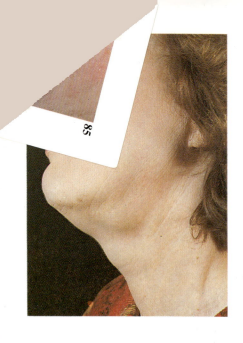

**87** This patient complained of swelling in the left sub-mandibular region made worse on eating and drinking.
(a) What is the probable diagnosis?
(b) What investigation is necessary to confirm this diagnosis?
(c) What treatment may be necessary?

**88** (a) What lesion is apparent on this patient's right vocal cord?
(b) What is the probable diagnosis?
(c) What treatment is necessary?

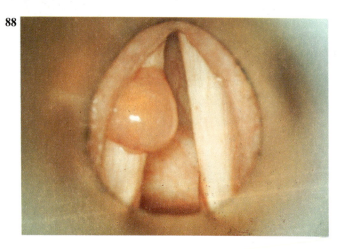

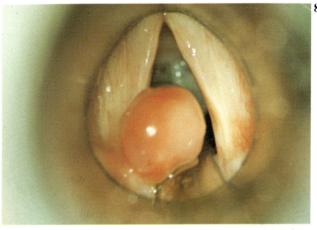

**89** This pedunculated lesion arises from the posterior aspect of the left vocal cord. This lesion, associated with hoarseness, presented four weeks after an operation for an abdominal procedure.
(a) What is the probable diagnosis?
(b) What is the treatment?
(c) Is the management of this problem usually straightforward?

**90** (a) What nasal deformity is apparent in this patient?
(b) There is also pain and tenderness over the larynx and the cartilage of the ear pinna has become soft and flaccid. What is the diagnosis?

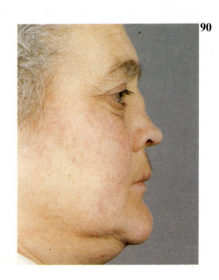

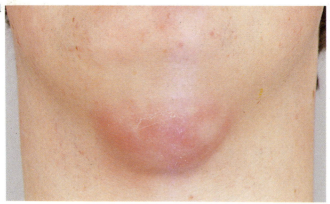

**91** This tender mid-line neck swelling recurred four months after previous surgery to the neck.
(a) What is the probable diagnosis?
(b) What step may well have been overlooked in the previous operation?

**92** (a) What abnormality does examination of the anterior nares demonstrate?
(b) What treatment is necessary for this condition?
(c) What are the possible complications of this treatment?

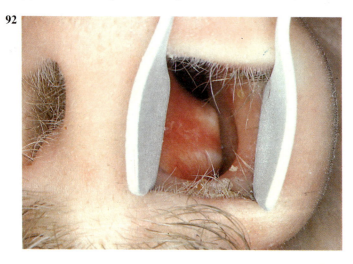

**93** (a) What operation has this patient undergone?
(b) The complaint, four days post-operatively, is of extreme discomfort and irritation in the region of the pinna — what signs are apparent?
(c) What is the probable diagnosis?

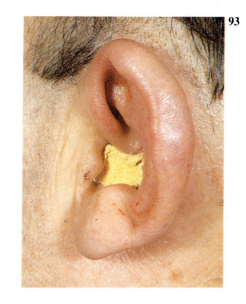

**94** (a) What bone is being demonstrated?
(b) What is its 'claim to fame' in the body?
(c) What condition specifically affects this bone causing hearing loss?
(d) What part of this bone is involved in this condition?

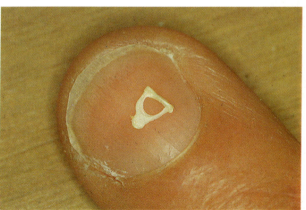

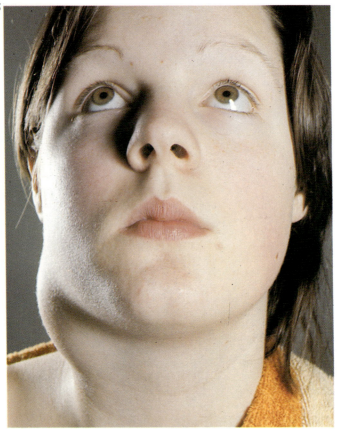

**95** This young girl presented with a large cystic swelling of four months' duration on the right side of the neck, which was gradually increasing in size.
(a) What diagnosis is suggested by the site of this swelling?
(b) What is the treatment?

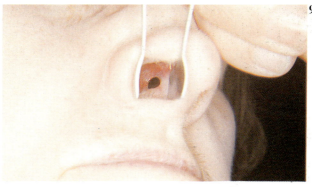

**96** (a) What abnormality does examination of the anterior nares demonstrate?
(b) What are the possible causes?
(c) What are the usual symptoms?
(d) Is treatment straightforward?

**97** This patient dislikes the prominent swelling of the medial aspect of the left nasal vestibule.
(a) What structures are involved?
(b) What muscle, on smiling, tends to accentuate these prominences?

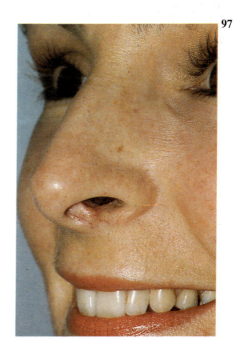

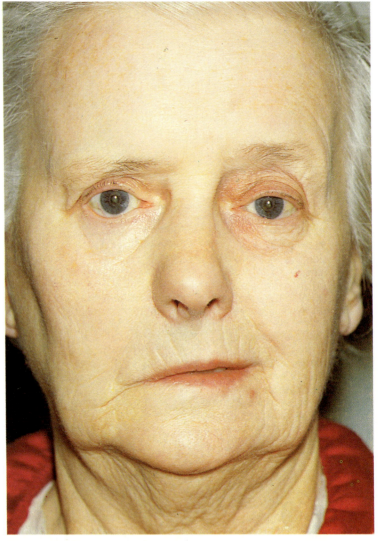

**98** This elderly patient, with a long past history of right otorrhoea and hearing loss, presented with some right ear pain and bleeding.
(a) What abnormality does this photograph demonstrate?
(b) What are the probable diagnoses?

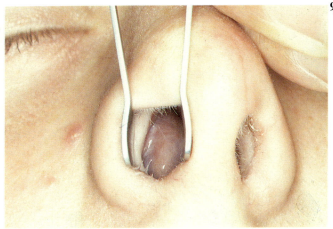

**99** A complaint of nasal obstruction, more marked on the right side, is associated with this finding on examination of the anterior nares.
(a) What structure is demonstrated?
(b) What are the characteristics of this structure?
(c) What is the probable diagnosis and treatment?

**100** (a) What are the characteristics of this tender, superficial ulcer of one day's duration?
(b) What is the diagnosis?
(c) What is the prognosis?
(d) What is the treatment?

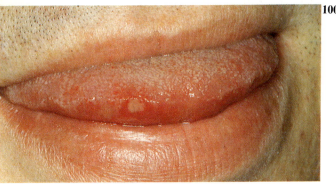

100

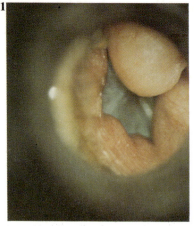

**101** A view of the tympanic membrane is occluded by these bony, hard, smooth swellings in the deep meatus.
(a) What is the diagnosis?
(b) Which occupation predisposes to their development?
(c) What is the management?

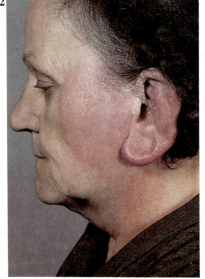

**102** This middle-aged woman presented with a hot, painful erythema surrounding the left ear. A flu-like illness with some discomfort in the ear preceded this episode.
(a) What is characteristic of this erythema of the cheek?
(b) What is the diagnosis?
(c) What condition probably triggered this infection?
(d) What is the treatment and prognosis?

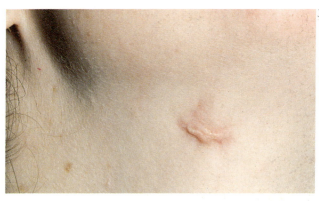

**103** A sebaceous cyst was removed from this patient's neck. The skin was sutured meticulously but the poor scar is apparent.
(a) What has almost certainly predisposed to this poor healing?
(b) Are sebaceous cysts on the face and neck straightforward to excise and enucleate?

**104** Examination of the left nares in a patient complaining of nasal obstruction showed a nasal polyp.
(a) What are the characteristics of this polyp?
(b) What are the possible diagnoses?
(c) What is the management?

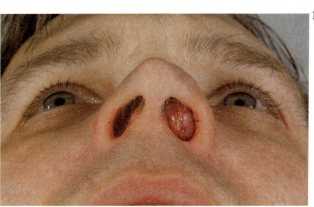

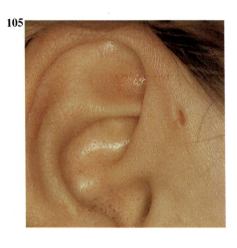

**105** Intermittent discharge with occasional swelling in front of the right ear were the presenting problems.
(a) What is the diagnosis?
(b) What is the management?
(c) Is the management simple and straightforward?

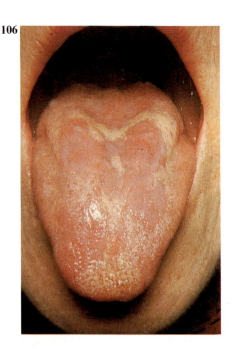

**106** This patient was concerned about these smooth pink areas over the dorsum of the tongue, which were otherwise symptom free.
(a) What is the diagnosis?
(b) What is the treatment?
(c) What are the complications?

**107** (a) What is this congenital auricular abnormality?
(b) From which tubercles does the pinna develop?
(c) What is the treatment?

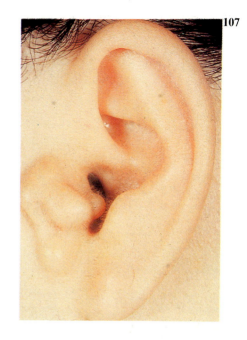

**108** (a) What pathology is apparent on examination of the oropharynx?
(b) What are the probable symptoms?

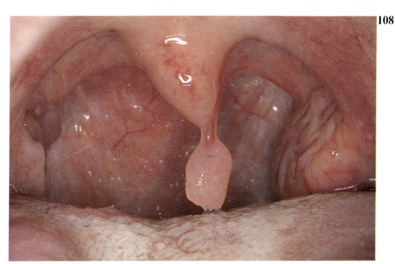

**109**

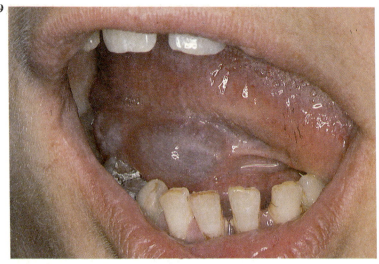

**109** (a) What are the characteristics of this swelling in the floor of the mouth?
(b) What is the diagnosis?
(c) What is the treatment?

**110**

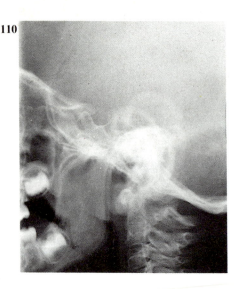

**110** (a)What abnormality does this lateral x-ray of a child's post-nasal space and pharynx show?
(b) What is the cause of this appearance?
(c) What will be one of the most predominant symptoms?

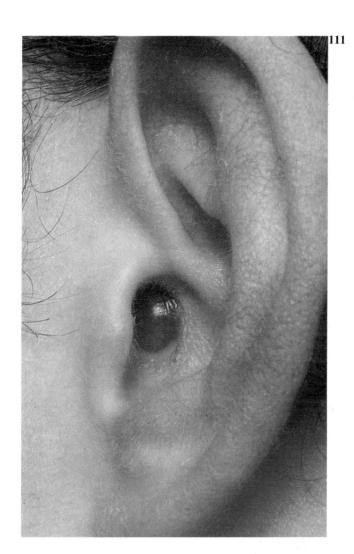

**111** This swelling apparent at the orifice of the left external auditory meatus was associated with a long past history of left ear discharge.
(a) What is the diagnosis?
(b) What is the probable underlying aural condition?
(c) What treatment is required?

**112**

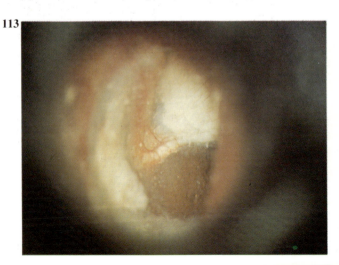

**112** This patient complained of a protruberance on the margin of the pinna.
(a) Which site of the pinna is this lesion on?
(b) Whose name is attached to this particular abnormality?
(c) Did this person initially describe the abnormality?

**113** (a) What abnormality does this right tympanic membrane show?
(b) Are these related to previous aural disease?

**113**

**114** During an aeroplane descent, severe pain was felt in the ear.
(a) What factors may predispose to this?
(b) What signs can be seen in the tympanic membrane?
(c) What is the prognosis?

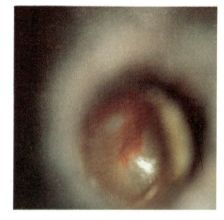

**115** This young patient complained of a sensation of pressure or discomfort, as if a foreign body had lodged in the region of the cricoid. There is no history suggestive of an impacted foreign body.
(a) What is the probable diagnosis?
(b) What direct question always confirms this diagnosis?
(c) What investigation is necessary?

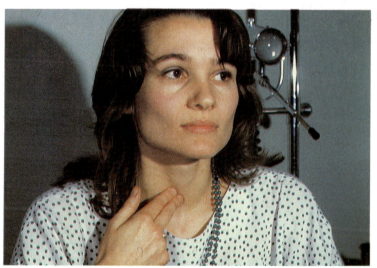

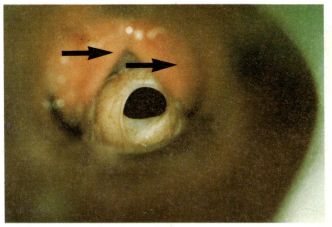

**116** A narrowing of the upper trachea is seen on direct laryngoscopy. The vocal cords (arrowed) are proximal and reddened.
(a) What is this tracheal narrowing?
(b) Name two causes.

**117** (a) What is this x-ray?
(b) What pathology is shown?
(c) What factors may underly this pathology?

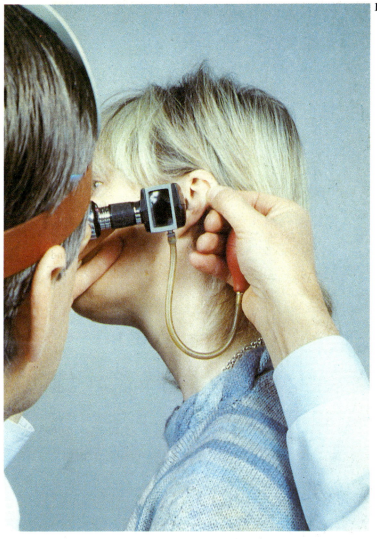

**118** (a) What instrument is being used in this ear examination?
(b) What technique is employed?
(c) In which conditions is this procedure helpful to diagnosis?

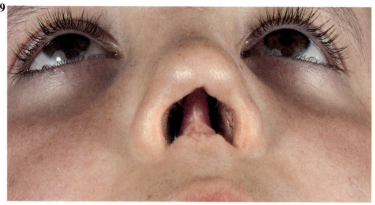

**119** (a) On which part of the nose does this 12-year-old boy have a defect?
(b) Is reconstruction of this part of the nose straightforward?
(c) What are the possible reconstruction techniques?

**120** This young man, with a history of recent injury to the nose, vigorously blew his nose and was alarmed to find immediate swelling of the soft tissues around the left eye which initially closed the eye.
(a) What is the probable diagnosis?
(b) What predisposed to this condition?
(c) What is felt on palpation?

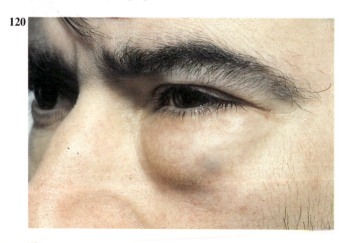

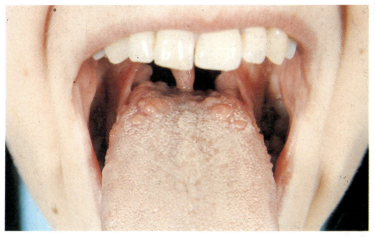

**121** On protrusion of the tongue, this patient was alarmed to see stud-like swellings on the base of the tongue.
(a) What are these structures?
(b) What is the nerve supply?
(c) What is the phylogenetic significance of this nerve supply?

**122** This young West Indian noticed a cystic non-tender swelling at the base of the nose on the left side which was gradually increasing in size.
(a) What are the characteristics of this swelling?
(b) What is the spot-diagnosis?
(c) What is the treatment?

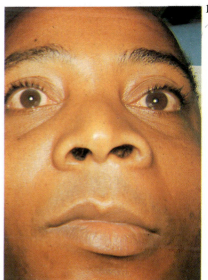

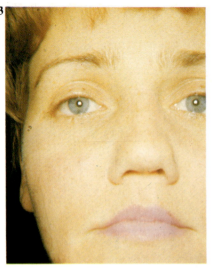

**123** (a) What is abnormal about the anatomy of this nose?
(b) What condition predisposes to this structure?

**124** A common cold had persisted for more than five days. Examination of the anterior nares showed this purulent exudate.
(a) What is the probable diagnosis?
(b) What other symptoms may be present?
(c) What investigations may be helpful in diagnosis and management?
(d) What is the treatment?

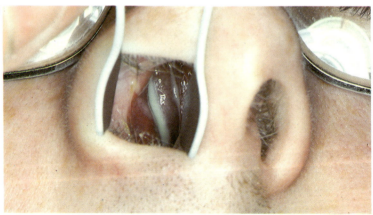

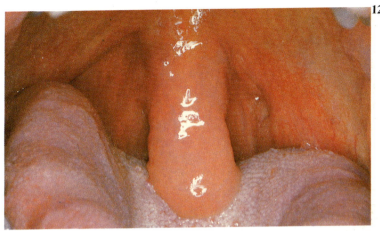

**125** (a) What abnormality is evident on examination of this oropharynx?
(b) What symptoms may accompany this finding?
(c) What investigations may be necessary?
(d) What treatment may be indicated?


**126** This painful oral ulcer had been present for two days and there was a past history of similar ulcers or crops of ulcers.
(a) What is the diagnosis?
(b) What is the aetiology?
(c) What is the treatment?

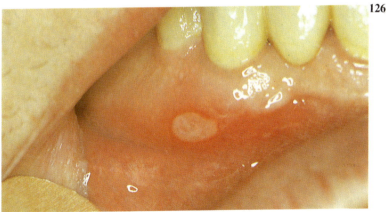

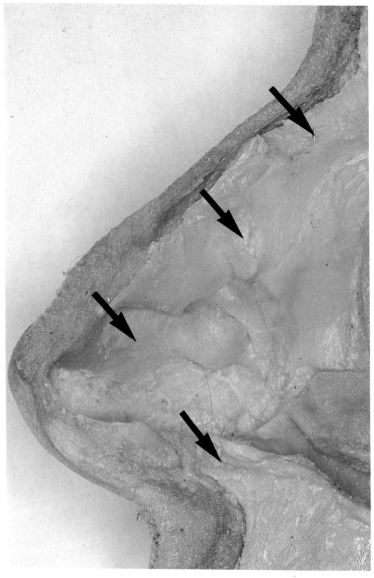

**127** What structures are arrowed in this cadaver dissection of the nose?

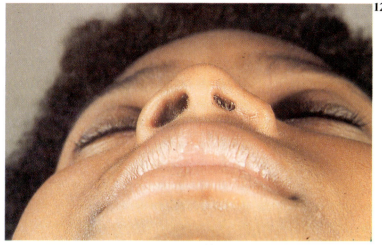

**128** This 12-year-old boy gave a history of left epistaxis and subsequent treatment for control of bleeding.
(a) What abnormality is now apparent on examination?
(b) What treatment could possibly have lead to this situation?
(c) What treatments are available to control epistaxis?

**129** Following a blow to the right ear, this young man presented with swelling of the upper part of the pinna.
(a) What is the diagnosis?
(b) What is the treatment?
(c) What is the prognosis?

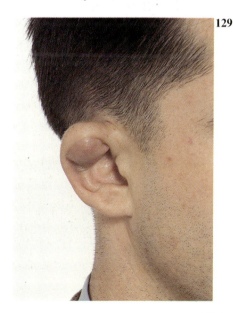

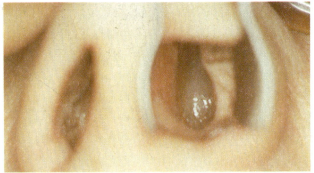

**130** This patient complained of nasal obstruction. On examination, a swelling in the left nasal fossa was apparent.
(a) What are the characteristics of this swelling?
(b) What is the diagnosis?
(c) What investigation may be necessary?
(d) What is the treatment?

**131** Numerous leashes of blood vessels were apparent, involving the mucosa of Little's area of the nose. The remaining septal mucosa was similarly involved. This patient complained of long-standing recurrent epistaxis.
(a) What is the diagnosis?
(b) What other findings may be seen on examination?
(c) What are possible treatments?

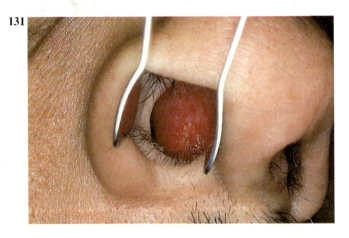

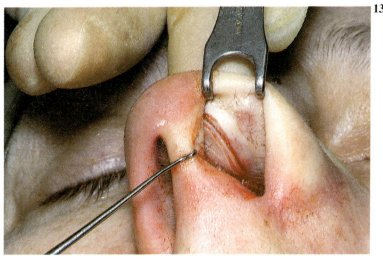

**132** An intra nasal incision has been made in the nasal vestibule.
(a) Which cartilage has been incised?
(b) In which operation is this incision frequently employed?

**133** (a) What is the anatomical deformity in the prominent or 'bat' ear?
(b) At what age is correction usually advised?

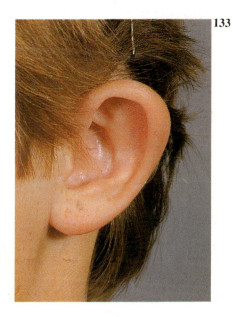

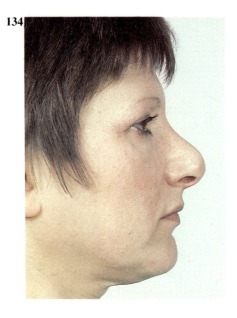

**134** (a) What type of nasal surgery has this patient undergone?

(b) What is the term commonly used to describe this nasal appearance?

(c) What two surgical faults predispose to this appearance?

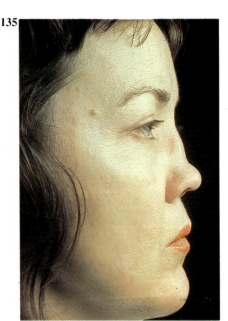

**135** (a) What term is applied to this nasal deformity?

(b) Name two complications of nasal trauma that may lead to this deformity.

(c) Name three chronic inflammatory conditions which may cause this condition.

**136** (a) What is this x-ray?
(b) What abnormalities are evident?
(c) Name two conditions that may cause this problem.
(d) Which two symptoms would this be associated with?

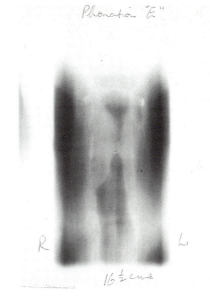

**137** (a) What abnormality is present?
(b) What is the cause?
(c) What may neck palpation reveal?

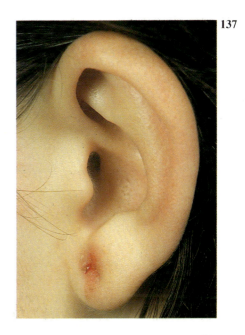

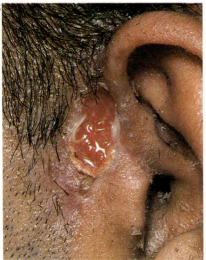

**138** (a) What is the cause of recurrent swelling and discharge with loss of skin in this site?
(b) What may be relevant in the past history?
(c) What is the treatment?

**139** Following a middle ear operation, this patient complained of a metallic taste and some dryness in the mouth.
(a) What abnormality is apparent on examination of this tongue?
(b) What middle ear nerve has been damaged to cause the symptoms and the changes apparent on this tongue?
(c) What other structures are supplied by this nerve?

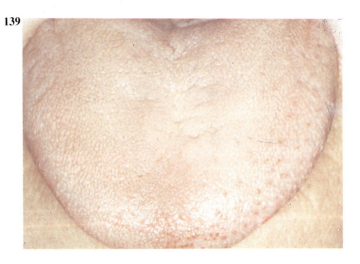

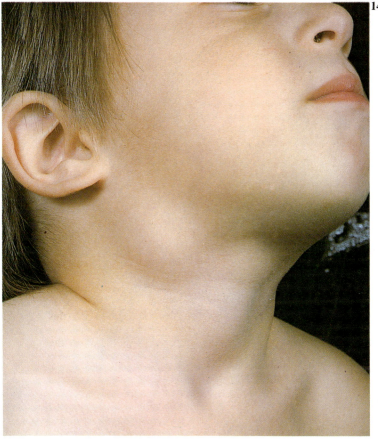

**140** This five-year-old boy had a swelling of three days' duration, apparent on the neck, which was tender to palpation. Recurrent episodes of malaise and fever were also reported.
(a) What lymph node lies in this site?
(b) What would examination of the oropharynx probably reveal?

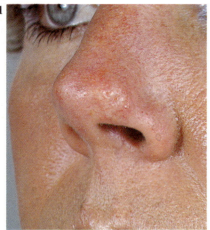

**141** An area of thickened and irregular skin, overlying the left side of the tip of the nose, had been present for three years. It had been concealed with cosmetics.
(a) What is the probable diagnosis?
(b) What investigations are necessary?
(c) What treatments are possible?

**142** (a) What is apparent on examination of this nasal vestibule?
(b) What site is involved?
(c) What is the probable cause and predisposing factor?

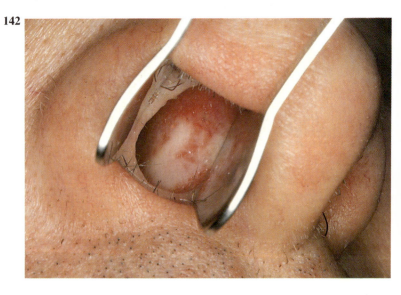

**143** Extreme itching and irritation of the ear was associated with discharge.
(a) What is the diagnosis?
(b) What investigation may be helpful?
(c) What direct question may give a further clue to the aetiology?

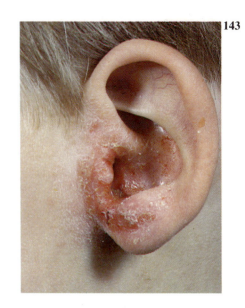

**144** This bony-hard palatal swelling was a chance-finding on dental examination.
(a) What is the diagnosis?
(b) What are the characteristics?
(c) What is the treatment?

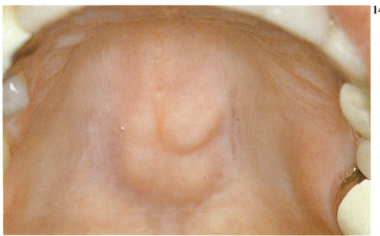

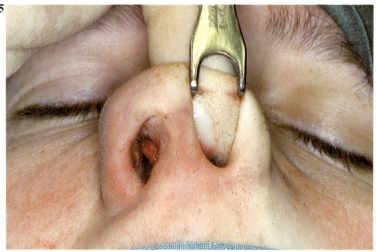

**145** (a) The lateral aspect of the nasal vestibule is exposed, delineating the margin of which structure?
(b) In what operation may this structure need modification?

**146** (a) What structure is demonstrated and has been surgically exposed?
(b) What use may be made of this material?

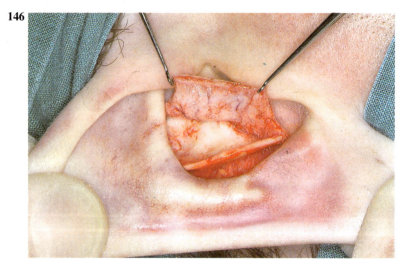

147A

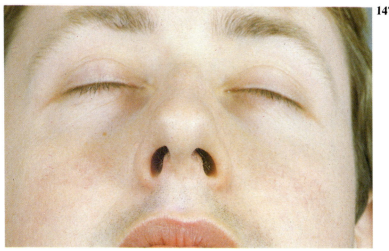

147B

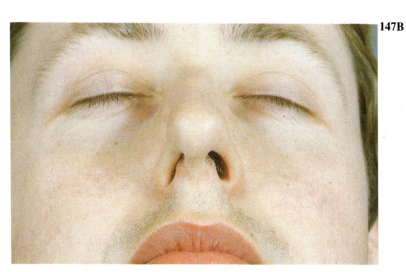

**147** (a) On gentle inspiration, what abnormality is apparent in this patient's nares?
(b) Is the situation demonstrated here common?
(c) What solutions may be available?

**148**

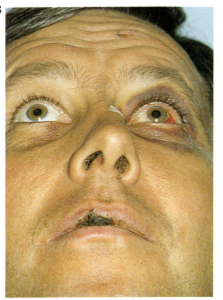

**148** This patient had suffered a recent injury to the right side of the nose with a fist.
(a) What nasal and ophthalmic abnormalities are apparent?
(b) There is also a complaint of total nasal obstruction. What is the likely cause?
(c) Subsequent rhinorrhoea may be suggestive of what complication?

**149**

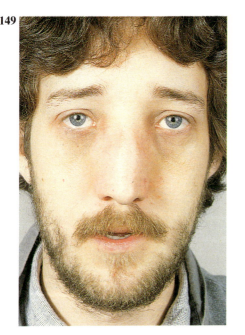

**149** (a) What abnormality is apparent on examination of this patient's nose?
(b) There is marked nasal obstruction and a history of many past operations: what is the probable diagnosis?

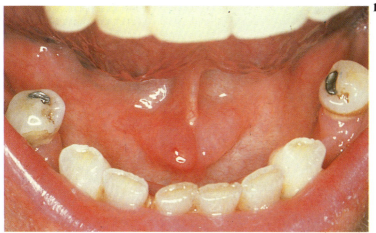

**150** Intermittent swelling of the neck when eating, was the presenting complaint of this patient.
(a) What does examination of the floor of the mouth show?
(b) What is the diagnosis?
(c) What is the treatment?

**151**

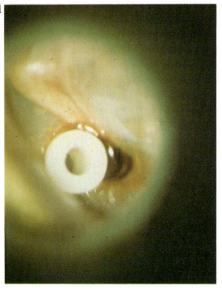

**151** A grommet is in place in this tympanic membrane.
(a) For which condition are these inserted?
(b) Does audiometry post-operatively show normal hearing or a slight degree of conductive hearing loss?
(c) As a rule, do grommets extrude in: three months, six months, or over nine months?
(d) Is the insertion of grommets a common operation?

**152**

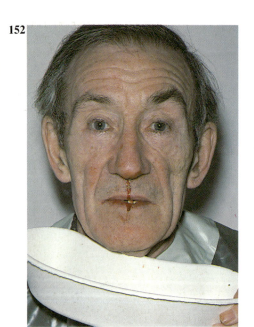

**152** This patient presented with spontaneous epistaxis.
(a) Is he best managed initially sitting up or lying down?
(b) What is the simplest first measure of controlling bleeding?
(c) From which site do most nose bleeds occur?
(d) Which vessels supply this site?

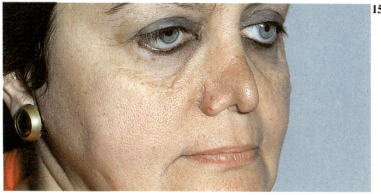

**153** (a) What is the significant, conspicuous abnormality of this patient's nose?
(b) What symptom, other than a dislike of the appearance, will be present?
(c) What may have predisposed to this condition?
(d) What management is possible?

**154** (a) What are the characteristics of the lesion apparent on this patient's chin?
(b) What examination and investigation may lead to the diagnosis?
(c) What is the probable diagnosis?

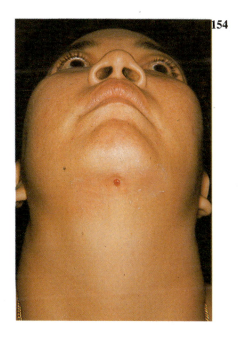

**155** (a) What abnormality is apparent in this tympanic membrane?
(b) What characteristic may be revealed by careful observation with the otoscope?
(c) What is the probable diagnosis?

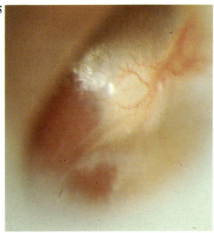

**156** (a) What x-ray is this?
(b) What are the obvious abnormalities?
(c) What may have led to this situation?

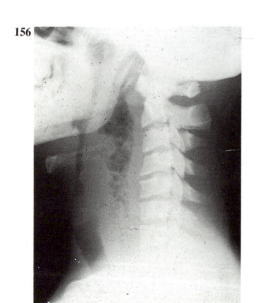

**157** (a) What does this barium swallow x-ray demonstrate?
(b) With what symptoms referable to swallowing may this problem be associated?
(c) What chest symptoms and signs may be associated?

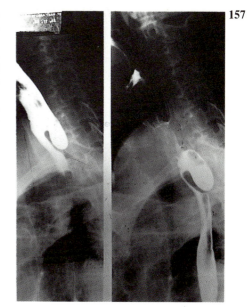

**158** (a) What abnormality is apparent on these tonsils?
(b) What symptoms are associated?
(c) What is the treatment?

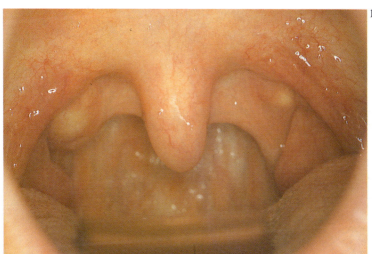

**159**

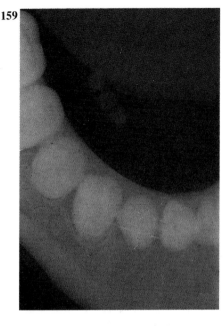

**159** An intraoral x-ray showing the floor of the mouth.
(a) What abnormality does this x-ray demonstrate?
(b) What symptoms would be associated?
(c) What treatment may be effective?

**160**

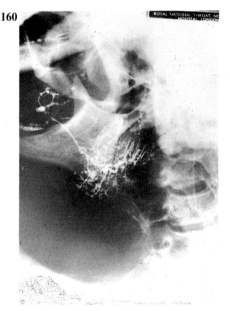

**160** (a) What x-ray is this?
(b) Is this a common investigation?
(c) What abnormality is demonstrated?

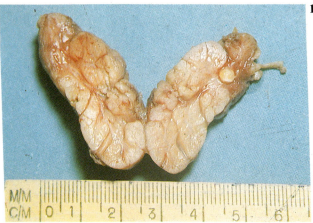

**161** This operative specimen demonstrates the submandibular gland and duct, with the submandibular gland having been opened.
(a) What abnormality is demonstrable?
(b) With what symptoms would this problem be associated?
(c) Why was excision of the gland necessary?

**162** A pink swelling laterally and a grey swelling more medially adjacent to the septum are apparent in the anterior nares. What are these structures and what characteristics of the more medial swelling make spot provisional diagnosis possible?

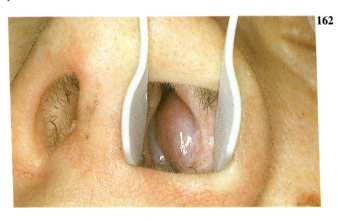

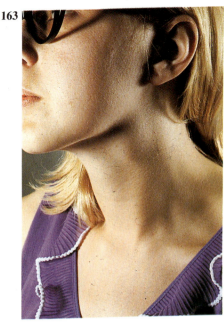

**163** (a) What are the characteristics of this neck swelling?
(b) What is the probable diagnosis?
(c) What treatment is necessary?
(d) What structure lies closely related to the deep surface of this swelling?

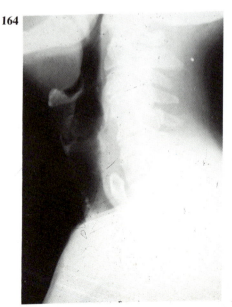

**164** (a) What is the abnormality seen in this lateral soft tissue x-ray of the cervical spine?
(b) What treatment will be necessary?
(c) What complication may arise?

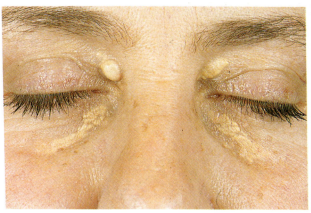

**165**

**165** (a) ·What condition affects this patient's eyes?
(b) What blood test should be carried out?
(c) What is the management?
(d) What is a possible complication?

**166** This adult presented with discomfort in the right side of his throat which had persisted after a severe sore throat eight weeks previously and had settled with a course of antibiotics.
(a) What are the findings?
(b) What are the possible diagnoses?
(c) What is the management?

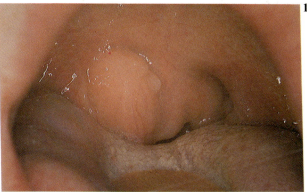

**166**

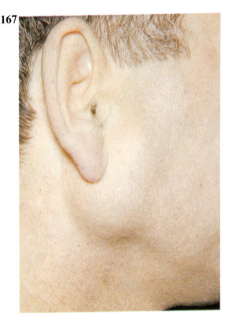

**167** This cheek/neck swelling was slow-growing and non-tender.
(a) What is the probable diagnosis?
(b) What cranial nerve should be checked?
(c) What treatment is usually necessary?

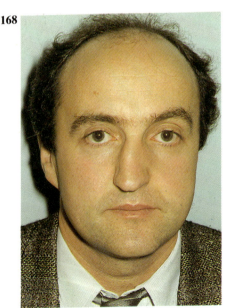

**168** Six months after nasal injury, this patient presented complaining of marked external deviation of the nose.
(a) What other nasal symptom is likely to be present?
(b) What treatment may be necessary?

**169** Intermittent, scanty bleeding from this facial ulcer, slowly increasing in size over two years, was the presentation of this lesion.
(a) What is the probable diagnosis?
(b) What are the possible treatments?
(c) What is the prognosis?

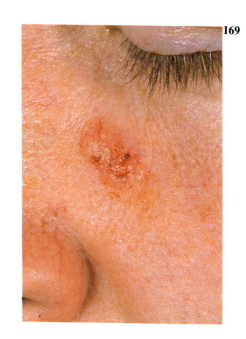

**170** (a) What is the possible cause of this lesion on the lobule of the ear?
(b) What will the histology show?

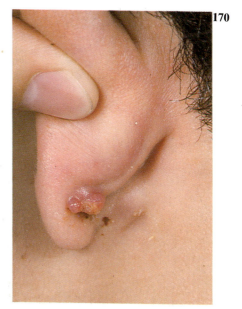

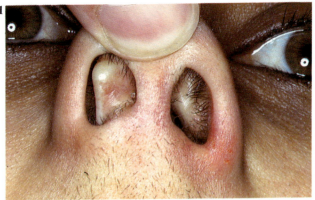

**171** A complaint of bilateral nasal obstruction, more marked on the right side, was the presenting symptom of this patient.
(a) What is the obvious abnormality on examination of the anterior nares?
(b) What direct question may reveal the cause of this abnormality?
(c) What is the management?

**172** (a) What abnormality does examination of the anterior nares in this patient show?
(b) What may more posterior examination of the nasal fossae reveal?
(c) Is this always an isolated condition?

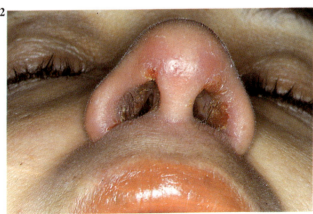

**173** (a) This photograph was taken during surgical excision of a submandibular gland. Two structures (arrowed) are apparent in the submandibular triangle and are found closely related to the submandibular gland.
(a) What are the arrowed structures?
(b) What more superficial nerve is at risk during excision of the submandibular gland?
(c) What deformity of the face ensues if this nerve is damaged?

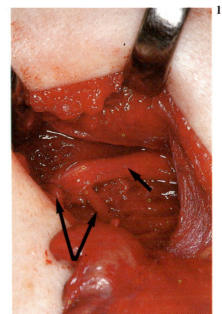

**174** (a) What abnormality is presented by this ten-year-old's anterior nares?
(b) What symptoms are probable?
(c) What is the possible management?

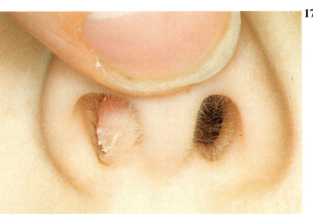

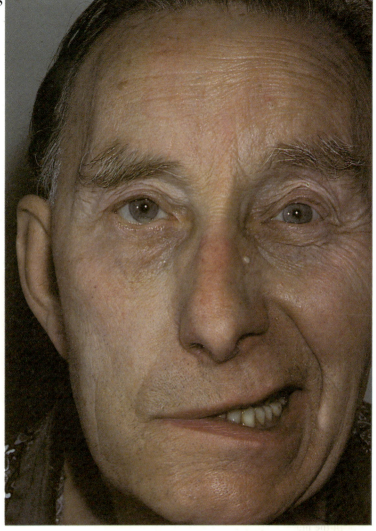

**175** (a) What is the obvious abnormality on examination of this patient's face?
(b) What is the common diagnosis?
(c) What symptoms may precede this problem?
(d) What is the prognosis and management?

# ANSWERS

**1** (a) Little's area (or Kiesselbach's plexus).
(b) It is the commonest site of epistaxis.
(c) Terminal branches of the superior labial artery, the sphenopalatine artery, the anterior superior dental artery, the maxillary artery.

**2** (a) The maxillary division of the Vth cranial nerve.
(b) Herpes zoster.

**3** (a) Nasal foreign body.
(b) Right maxillary sinusitis with purulent nasal discharge causing the vestibulitis.

**4** (a) Deviated nasal septum. The cartilage has been dislocated off the maxillary crest into the right nasal fossa.
(b) Gentle palpation will confirm this to be a firm swelling and exclude the possibility of a nasal polyp.

**5** (a) A left nasal polyp.
(b) A simple nasal polyp does not bleed and the appearance of the surface of the polyp is not entirely smooth and opalescent. Therefore, the histology must be checked (as with all nasal polyps) to exclude the possibility of malignancy.

**6** (a) A pharyngo- or laryngocele.
(b) This tends to occur in wind-instrument players.

**7** Mumps with abscess development overlying the submandibular gland. Dental abscess.

**8** (a) A thyroglossal cyst with recurrent infection.
(b) A past history of excision of a neck swelling (in which the body of the hyoid bone has not been included), makes the diagnosis of a thyroglossal cyst virtually certain.

**9** (a) A bone graft taken from the iliac crest has been used to supplement the nasal bones.
(b) A saddle deformity usually resulting from trauma or chronic inflammatory disease.
(c) One long-term problem with iliac bone graft is resorbtion and loss of the graft.

**10** (a) The cartilagenous nasal septum has been exposed by an incision through the mucosa and muco-perichondrium.
(b) An operation to correct deviation of the nasal septum (an SMR or septoplasty) is being performed.

**11** (a) Surgical emphysema.
(b) A fracture has occurred through the lamina papyracia. On blowing the nose, air tracks into the orbit via the ethmoid sinus. There is a subconjunctival haematoma and also a possible fracture of the floor of the orbit, but other eye injuries should be excluded.

**12** (a) The commonest site for carcinoma of the larynx is on the vocal cord (glottic 70%, supraglottic 20%, subglottic 10%).
(b) The prognosis is excellent for early glottic carcinoma.
(c) Radiotherapy.

**13** (a) Binder's syndrome.
(b) A rhinoplasty with grafting in the region of the anterior nasal spine and premaxilla.

**14** (a) Nasal vestibulitis with a change of the nasal mucus membrane to squamous epithelium with leucoplakia.
(b) This is caused by rubbing or irritating the nose over a period of years — excessive nose cleaning or picking of the nose.
(c) The patient should be asked if he uses cocaine: this may set up a vestibulitis.

**15** (a) The epistaxis is related to vessels at the margin of a septal perforation.
(b) Septal perforations may occur in those who sniff cocaine. They also occur in obsessional nose pickers or those who work with chrome. A vestibulitis is set up, predisposing to a septal perforation. (See **96**.)

**16** (a) An antrochoanal polyp.
(b) A sinus x-ray will reveal complete opacity of the antrum on that side and a soft tissue swelling characteristic of this type of polyp will be seen in the post-nasal space.
(c) Antral proof puncture will reveal straw-coloured fluid.

**17** (a) Snail-track ulcers of secondary syphilis.
(b) The VDRL is positive, and the throat microscopy will reveal spirochaetes.

**18** (a) Relapsing polychondritis.
(b) In this condition the inflammatory changes in the cartilage involve particularly the ear and the larynx but also the septum (causing a saddle deformity). Cartilage elsewhere in the body becomes involved. A biopsy of the ear cartilage reveals histology diagnostic of this condition.

**19** (a) A perichondritis.
(b) Pseudomonas pyocyaneus. In this condition a diffuse inflammation, associated with severe pain, infiltrates the cartilage of the pinna. If this is not treated vigorously with appropriate antibiotics and possible surgical drainage, gross deformity of the pinna, as demonstrated here, results.

**20** (a) Enlarged tonsils and adenoids causing upper respiratory tract obstruction.
(b) Sleep studies are necessary to exclude obstructive sleep apnoea.
(c) It is probable that interference with Eustachian tube function has caused glue ear accounting for the hearing loss.
(d) Mouth breathing and indrawing of the intercostal muscles. Also pectus excavatum.

**21** (a) A skin infiltration involving the tip of the nose and upper lip, characteristic of pernio.
(b) The probable diagnosis is sarcoid.

**22** (a) A projection in the lateral wall of the right nasal vestibule which may cause limitation of airway on that side.
(b) This projection is occasionally caused by a prominent and projecting lateral crus of the alar cartilage.

**23** This is the normal appearance of the fauces following tonsillectomy and the patient can be reassured.

**24** (a) Glomus jugulare tumour accounting for the conductive hearing loss and pulsating tinnitus.
(b) The cranial nerves involved are those emerging through the jugular foramen and the near-by anterior condular foramen. The IX, X and XI emerge through the jugular foramen, and the XII (left hypoglossal nerve) which is damaged in this case causing the tongue changes, emerges through the anterior condylar foramen. Glomus jugulare tumours extend from the floor of the middle ear along the base of the skull to involve these structures.

**25** A prolapse, or particularly prominent and medially placed lateral crus of the alar cartilage. Incision lines are seen at the alar bases and narrowing of the alae has been carried out by a Weir's incision during a rhinoplasty operation. This leads, on occasions, to narrowing of the nasal vestibule limiting the airway.

**26** (a) Examination shows that the tonsil itself is not enlarged but pushed medially by a parapharyngeal swelling.
(b) The diagnosis therefore is a pleomorphic adenoma of the parotid gland, pushing the tonsil medially and simulating tonsil enlargement.

**27** (a) A left orbital proptosis is apparent (best confirmed by examination from above).
(b) The orbit is displaced laterally and inferiorly and this appearance is usually caused by a fronto-ethmoidal mucocele.
(c) A history of previous nasal surgery in the region of the ethmoids is not uncommon with mucoceles.

**28** (a) Basal cell carcinoma.
(b) Biopsy.
(c) Excision with full thickness skin graft.

**29** (a) The tonsils show a characteristic white/yellow membrane.
(b) The membrane is characteristic of infectious mononucleosis (glandular fever).
(c) Ampicillin is to be avoided in this condition for there is hypersensitivity and an uncomfortable skin urticaria will develop.

**30** (a) There is a clot in the left tonsillar fossa (the normal appearance of the fossa at this stage is illustrated at **23**).
(b) The appearance represents secondary infection.
(c) Antibiotics and possible admission to hospital for observation and blood transfusion, if the bleeding is severe or persists. It is sometimes but not always, helpful to remove the clot from the tonsillar fossa.

**31** (a) A septal deviation to the left.
(b) The quadrilateral septal cartilage has been dislocated off the maxillary crest.
(c) A septoplasty or submucous resection (SMR).

**32** (a) An aphthous ulcer.
(b) The endo-tracheal tube when inserted orally may have caused a slight abrasion to the soft palate.
(c) A past history of oral aphthous ulceration. Minor trauma is a known trigger for aphthous ulcers in those who are susceptible.

**33** (a) Sinus x-rays (Townes view) demonstrating the maxillary sinuses.
(b) **B** is a tilted view to demonstrate that the lines apparent in **A** are definitely fluid levels.
(c) Fluid in the antra as demonstrated here may occur with maxillary sinusitis, nasal allergy or occasionally haematoma following injury.

**34** (a) Reconstruction of the ear canal and ossicles to restore the hearing in a one-sided meatal atresia is not adviseable in childhood in the presence of a normal other ear.
(b) Pinna reconstruction requires many surgical stages and is not straightforward. The alternatives are to leave alone or consider an osseo-integrated prosthesis.

**35** (a) The lymph nodes in the posterior triangle of the neck.
(b) Tuberculosis is the commonest chronic inflammatory condition giving rise to this appearance.

**36** (a) Angular stomatitis.
(b) Glossitis and dysphagia due to a cricopharyngeal web or spasm.
(c) The Plummer-Vinson syndrome (or Paterson-Brown-Kelly syndrome). The possible long-term complication is of a post-cricoid carcinoma.

**37** (a) Sebaceous cyst.
(b) The punctum is just apparent on close examination. In the absence of a punctum, a parotid swelling or an enlarged parotid lymph node are the differential diagnoses.

**38** The x-ray on the left which shows the post-nasal space has been taken obliquely. The angles of the mandible show that this is not a true lateral x-ray. The apparent occlusion of the postnasal space by bulk of adenoids is therefore an artefact. The lateral x-ray to show the bulk of adenoid tissue is reliable only if the x-ray is a true lateral.

**39** Aneurysm of the left internal carotid artery.

**40** (a) The lesion is almost certainly a neoplasm.
(b) A benign lesion of this type presenting with bleeding could well be a haemangioma. A malignant nasal polyp is the other possibility. The site of origin proved to be from Little's area and this is in fact a septal haemangioma (bleeding polypus of the septum).
(c) Management of this lesion involves establishing the site of origin and then proceeding either to a biopsy or a biopsy excision.

**41** (a) Rhinolith.
(b) These are usually the result of a calcarious deposit forming around a long-standing foreign body.
(c) An increase in size and very firm impaction in the nasal fossa, so that erosion of the floor or lateral wall of the nose may occur. Large rhinoliths are therefore not easy to remove.

**42** The appearance and cervical lymphadenopathy are characteristic of a metal dermatitis related to earrings.

**43** (a) This is a laryngeal tomogram.
(b) An extensive subglottic stenosis with narrowing of the airway below the vocal cords is apparent.

**44** A pneumatic otoscope. Air is gently inflated against the drum and this membrane is seen to move. (See illustration **118**.)

**45** (a) 'Malignant' otitis externa.
(b) Biopsy will reveal simple granulation tissue.
(c) The organism cultured will be *Pseudomonas pyocyaneus*.

**46** (a) Transillumination of the maxillary sinuses. A bright light is placed in the patient's mouth in a darkened room.
(b) There is lack of transillumination of the right maxillary sinus.
(c) This appearance could be given by a right maxillary sinusitis or by a lesion occluding the right antrum such as a neoplasm.
(d) Transillumination, although an out-dated investigation, is of interest in cysts involving the maxillary sinus which transilluminate very brightly. It is also of interest to see whether a maxillary sinusitis is resolving in the absence of availability of good x-rays.

**47** (a) Examination shows an indurated ulcerated lesion with a hyperaemic margin involving the floor of the left nasal vestibule.
(b) A biopsy will be necessary for diagnosis.
(c) The clinical appearance of this lesion is that of a squamous (or possibly basal cell) carcinoma.

**48** (a) Keratosis pharyngeus.
(b) No treatment is necessary unless there is an associated history of tonsillitis.

**49** (a) Nasal bones, upper lateral cartilages, alar cartilages.
(b) External rhinoplasty.

**50** (a) Pharyngitis of fungal origin.
(b) *Candida albicans*.
(c) Lozenges containing an anti-fungal agent.

**51** (a) Mandibular division of the trigeminal nerve.
(b) Herpes zoster.

**52** Scleroma, syphilis or the uvulo-palatoplasty operation for snoring, give a palate of this appearance.

**53** (a) Keloid.
(b) Excision of a preauricular sinus.
(c) Recurrence after a simple excision of a keloid is invariable.

**54** (a) Rhinophyma.
(b) Shaving of the excess thick seborrhoeic skin.
(c) Biopsy is necessary if there is any suspicious area of skin, as basal or squamous cell carcinoma may occur within rhinophymata.

**55** (a) The swelling involves the tail of the right parotid gland.
(b) The probable diagnosis is a pleomorphic adenoma or a possible adenolymphoma (Warthin's tumour).
(c) For a pleomorphic adenoma, superficial parotidectomy is required.

**56** Mumps.

**57** (a) Bifid uvula.
(b) There are usually no symptoms and this is a chance finding.
(c) A submucosal palatal cleft may be apparent or palpable.

**58** (a) Unilateral enlargement of the left tonsil.
(b) This may be a chance finding of no significance, but if the asymmetry is gross and persistent, a lymphoma should be suspected. A chronic quinsy is another possibility. Careful examination to exclude medial displacement of the tonsil—simulating enlargement of the tonsil—is needed.
(c) The management required to exclude a tonsillar lymphoma is tonsillectomy/biopsy. A portion taken from the tonsil for biopsy may not give sufficient biopsy material for a definite diagnosis to be made.

**59** (a) Supratonsillar clefts—unusually large and obvious.
(b) Faetid tonsillar debris may collect in these clefts and cause an unpleasant taste in the mouth. It is possible that this may also cause halitosis.
(c) Tonsillectomy may be necessary.

**60** This patient has 'gagged' due to the pressure of the tongue depressor. This has caused the fauces to approximate and accentuate the 'large' appearance of the tonsils. The tonsils are however hyperaemic, and there is a complaint of sore throat with some fever, so that tonsillitis is an additional factor accounting for the tonsillar enlargement. It is not however as gross and as obstructing as it first appears on account of the gagging.

**61** (a) Parotid calculus impacted at the orifice of the parotid duct (Stensen's duct).
(b) Incision under local anaesthetic to remove any calculus.
(c) These calculi are uncommon and considerably less common than those occurring in the submandibular duct.

**62** (a) A short lingual frenulum—'tongue tie'.
(b) This degree of tongue tie usually only limits the ability to protrude the tongue. There is no interference with speech in most cases.
(c) No treatment is necessary in almost all cases but a very tight frenulum in which the speech production is altered requires division, or a Z-plasty.

**63** (a) Torus mandibularis.
(b) No treatment is required, for these are normally symptom-free and chance findings on examination.

**64** (a) Follicular tonsillitis.
(b) Throat swab for culture and sensitivity.
(c) Penicillin orally for 5-10 days.
(d) The differential diagnosis is infectious mononucleosis although the exudate is not characteristic of this condition (See **Q29**). If however there are other symptoms and signs to suggest infectious mononucleosis, amoxicillin is to be avoided because of hypersensitivity.

**65** (a) Keloid formation following ear piercing.
(b) A sebaceous cyst, if the lesion was soft and a punctum was apparent.
(c) The treatment is not straightforward: recurrence is invariable following simple excision of a keloid, although low-dose radiotherapy, triamcinolone injections, and 'pressure' earrings (which are probably the most effective present treatment) are amongst the modalities used to avoid recurrence.

**66** (a) Gouty tophus.
(b) Serum uric acid.

**67** (a) Helix.
(b) This is either: a neoplasm (a basal cell carcinoma if the history is long, or a squamous cell carcinoma with a shorter history) or a chronic inflammatory lesion involving the underlying cartilage with breakdown of the overlying skin (chondrodermatitis nodularis helicis chronicis).
(c) A wedge excision/biopsy is necessary.

**68** (a) Synechiae or adhesions.
(b) These may well follow nasal surgery in which incisions of the nasal mucosa are 'opposite' one another on the medial and lateral wall of the nasal vestibule.
(c) Division with an in-dwelling Silastic splint left *in situ* until epithelialisation occurs.

**69** (a) Deviation of the nasal septum in which the quadrilateral cartilage has been dislocated off the maxillary crest to lie transversely, partly obstructing the left anterior nares with obstruction of the right nasal fossa posteriorly.
(b) A septoplasty is required to reposition this septum into the mid-line and restore the airway.

**70** (a) Fronto-ethmoidal sinusitis.
(b) Sinus x-ray and possible sinus CT scan.
(c) Intensive antibiotic therapy—probably IV with hospital admission. Surgical drainage may be necessary if resolution is not rapid and complete, or if improvement does not take place within 24/48 hours.
(d) A frontal lobe abscess may account for the headache and should be excluded.

**71** (a) Nasal papillomas are common in this site.
(b) Either excision/biopsy or removal with a curette is necessary. If there is any suspicion of this being a keratoacanthoma or basal cell carcinoma, excision is preferable to curettage.

**72** (a) A pyogenic granuloma. This heals spontaneously in most cases.
(b) Biopsy is necessary if this lesion does not regress. Serology is necessary to exclude a luetic ulcer.

**73** (a) Bleeding from the right tonsil.
(b) Bleeding from the tonsil is a rare but potentially serious complication of a quinsy (bleeding quinsy). Bleeding may also occur from the tonsil with severe acute tonsillitis as in this instance. Self-induced traumatic tonsil bleeding is also a possible diagnosis and is to be excluded by direct questioning.

**74** (a) A basal or squamous cell carcinoma of the nasal vestibule.
(b) A biopsy.

**75** (a) Geniculate herpes (The Ramsay Hunt syndrome).
(b) A facial palsy and vertigo are frequently associated with the sensorineural hearing loss and herpes.

**76** (a) Submandibular calculus.
(b) Incision of the submandibular duct (Wharton's duct) overlying the calculus.
(c) If the submandibular calculus is solitary and placed near the orifice of the duct, this procedure is curative. If however, there are more calculi posteriorly or within the submandibular gland, excision of the submandibular gland is necessary.

**77** (a) This mid-line, or near mid-line, cystic neck swelling moves up and down on swallowing, demonstrating its attachment to the larynx.
(b) Thyroglossal cyst.
(c) Excision is necessary, including the removal of the body of the hyoid bone.
(d) Failure to remove the hyoid bone body will be followed by recurrence, for the thyroglossal duct remnant tracks behind the body of the hyoid bone.

**78** (a) A slit-like perforation of the tympanic membrane is demonstrated with some fresh blood. These are the characteristics of a *traumatic* perforation of the tympanic membrane.
(b) A direct blow to the ear—usually a slap with a hand or a possible direct puncture.
(c) No treatment is necessary, other than care to avoid letting water into the ear. (This may predispose to infection presenting as otorrhoea and necessitating antibiotics.) Care should also be taken to avoid a forcible Valsalva by the patient on blowing the nose.
(d) The prognosis is good, with healing within 6 weeks in most cases. The larger traumatic perforations, or those extending to the periphery of the drum, may not heal spontaneously.

**79** (a) The caloric test. In this case the nystagmus is being monitored by an electronystagmograph (electronystagmography) rather than by simple observation.
(b) This investigation is helpful in the diagnosis of Meniere's Disease and acoustic neuromas.
(c) This test is contraindicated in the presence of a tympanic membrane perforation, and in mastoid cavities.

**80** (a) This is the chorda tympani nerve lying in an inferior position and hence being more than usually obvious through the translucent tympanic membrane.
(b) This nerve carries the parasympathetic secretomotor fibres to the submandibular and sublingual salivary glands. This nerve also carries taste from the buds on the anterior two-thirds of the tongue excluding the circumvallate papillae.

**81** (a) An attic aural polyp.
(b) A chronic otitis media with probable cholesteatoma.
(c) Removal/biopsy of this aural polyp. Subsequent mastoid exploration and tympanoplasty will probably be necessary.

**82** (a) A grommet has been inserted in the tympanic membrane.
(b) A grommet is inserted for glue ear (serous or secretory otitis media).
(c) The grommet has become occluded with haematoma/exudate. Fluid

remains behind the drum and a hearing improvement has not taken place following the operation.

**83** (a) A central tympanic membrane perforation.
(b) This perforation is 'safe'—there is little likelihood of cholesteatoma.
(c) Otorrhoea with head colds or following swimming.
(d) A myringoplasty operation has an excellent possibility of sealing this type of perforation.

**84** (a) This is the positional test in which the head, when placed backwards and to one side, triggers vertigo, with an associated nystagmus that fatigues. The vertigo and nystagmus recur on sitting up.
(b) This test is diagnostic of benign paroxysmal positional vertigo.

**85** (a) These sclerae show a characteristic blue colour.
(b) A conductive hearing loss may be the presenting symptom. The stapes foot-plate is ankylosed, as in otosclerosis.
(c) Osteogenesis imperfecta tarda.

**86** (a) A large posterior tympanic membrane perforation with an area of tympanosclerosis in the anterior superior quadrant.
(b) The round window, promontory, stapedius, stapes and long process of the incus are apparent through the perforation. The handle of the malleus with the umbo and malleus lateral process can also be seen.

**87** (a) Submandibular gland calculus.
(b) X-rays of the submandibular gland and duct.
(c) No treatment may be necessary if the calculi are small and 'pass'. If the calculi or calculus is large and impacted anteriorly in the duct, incision of the duct with removal of the calculus is effective (see **76**). If the calculus is lodged more posteriorly or within the submandibular gland, excision of the submandibular gland is necessary.

**88** (a) A right vocal cord polyp.
(b) The appearance is that of a benign polyp—the surface is smooth without ulceration.
(c) Excision using a microlaryngoscopic technique.

**89** (a) Intubation granuloma overlying the vocal process of the arytenoid.
(b) Excision of this lesion from its narrow peduncle is required, or a laser excision may be used.
(c) Recurrence of these intubation granulomas is common.

**90** (a) A saddle deformity is demonstrated due to collapse of the nasal septal cartilage.
(b) The tenderness over the larynx is related to cartilaginous involvement of the larynx. The ear cartilage is also involved, along with the septal cartilage, in this condition of relapsing polychondritis.

**91** (a) Recurrent thyroglossal cyst with infection (see **77**).
(b) The cyst alone was excised. The body of the hyoid bone was left and recurrence of the cyst with infection has occurred. Revision surgery is necessary following antibiotic therapy.

**92** (a) A septal deviation with a low spur, in which the quadrilateral septal cartilage has dislocated off the maxillary crest, which is also deviated.
(b) A septoplasty or submucous resection (SMR) operation is necessary.
(c) Bleeding with septal haematoma or a septal perforation.

**93** (a) A mastoidectomy operation with a meatoplasty. The obvious enlarged 'square' meatus demonstrates that a technique to enlarge the orifice of the meatus has been carried out.
(b) The pinna is reddened and swollen with some vesiculation.
(c) The irritation suggests an allergy to the dressing. The yellow colour of this dressing is characteristic of iodoform which is used in some aural dressings.

**94** (a) The innermost of the ear ossicles — the stapes bone.
(b) This is the smallest bone in the body.
(c) Otosclerosis.
(d) The footplate of the stapes bone, which is ankylosed in the foramen ovale impeding ossicular movement and giving rise to a conductive hearing loss.

**95** (a) This swelling is situated between the upper third and lower two-thirds of the sterno-mastoid muscle and is half-concealed by the muscle. This is strongly suggestive of a branchial cyst.
(b) Excision.

**96** (a) A septal perforation.
(b) This type of perforation may follow trauma to the vestibule of the nose either by cautery on both sides or by digital self-interference. Cocaine sniffing may also be a cause. Septal perforation is also an occasional complication of septal surgery. Chrome workers may also develop vestibulitis leading to a septal perforation.
(c) A small perforation may cause whistling. The large perforations tend to crust and bleed giving rise to some nasal discomfort and a sensation of 'congestion'. Most perforations however are symptom-free.
(d) Surgical closure of these perforations by nasal mucosal flaps or composite grafts do not carry a very good prognosis with a high incidence of graft breakdown.

**97** (a) A dislocation of the caudal end of the septum is causing increased prominence of the base of the medial crus of the alar cartilage.
(b) The musculus depressor septi pulls downwards on the nasal tip on smiling, with some curling of the upper lip. This accentuates the prominence of the septal dislocation and prominent medial crus.

**98** (a) A right lower motor neurone facial palsy. Note the 'flat' forehead on the right side.
(b) A right chronic otitis media, possibly with cholesteatoma that has involved the facial nerve. The presence of bleeding from the ear is unusual with chronic otitis media and there is a possibility of a squamous cell carcinoma (which has a higher incidence in CSOM).

**99** (a) The inferior turbinate.
(b) The attachment of this swelling to the lateral wall of the nose is apparent so that this is almost certainly an enlargement of the right inferior turbinate rather than a nasal polyp. This turbinate is blue/grey and pale in colour.
(c) This is the characteristic appearance of a turbinate enlarged with allergic oedema — as in hay fever or nasal allergy. (This is not the grey opalescent

colour of a nasal polyp.) A corticosteroid nasal spray or drops may reduce the mucosal oedema. Surgery to reduce such a grossly large turbinate may be necessary.

**100** (a) It has a pale centre with a hyperaemic margin, without induration.
(b) This is characteristic of an aphthous ulcer.
(c) This will heal spontaneously in a matter of days. It may well have been triggered by trauma against the teeth in those who are susceptible to these common recurrent ulcers.
(d) There is no specific treatment, but a corticosteroid applied to the ulcer or used as a lozenge may reduce the pain and speed healing.

**101** (a) Aural osteoma or hyperostosis.
(b) These are seen in swimmers and are known as 'swimmer's osteomas'.
(c) In most cases no treatment is needed. It is extremely rare for these to become so large as to occlude the meatus although this can occur. Wax may impact beyond these osteomas and give rise to otitis externa. These complications and occlusion of the meatus, call for removal with the aural drill. They are not to be removed with an osteotome, as a fissure fracture through the osteoma may cause bleeding extending to the facial nerve and lead to facial paralysis.

**102** (a) The erythema is raised and has a well-defined margin.
(b) This appearance is characteristic of erysipelas.
(c) Infection through a fissure in the external auditory meatus where there is an otitis externa may well have triggered this erysipelas which involves the pinna as well as the cheek.
(d) The fever, malaise, pain and erythema all settle rapidly with penicillin.

**103** (a) It is almost certain that the sebaceous cyst ruptured during removal and that a portion was left behind, leading to healing by secondary intention and this ugly raised scar.
(b) Sebaceous cysts on the face and neck are difficult to excise and enucleate and require particular care to remove complete in 'one piece'. They are considerably more difficult to remove than cysts in the scalp and elsewhere. Great care therefore is required with face and neck sebaceous cyst excisions to avoid scarring.

**104** (a) A simple nasal polyp has a grey and opalescent surface. When however it is exposed at the nasal vestibule, the surface may well become red. Examination more posteriorly will show a grey surface.
(b) The probable diagnosis is that of an 'exposed' nasal polyp.
(c) A unilateral nasal polyp should arouse suspicion of possible malignancy and biopsy/excision is necessary.

**105** (a) A preauricular sinus. The site is constant and characteristic.
(b) Excision of the preauricular sinus.
(c) Excision of a preauricular sinus is not straightforward as the sinus tracks deeply and requires to be excised *in toto*. If a part is left behind, recurrent discharge invariably occurs with revision operation presenting more difficult problems. It is often helpful to delineate the tract of these preauricular sinuses with an injection of a dye pre-operatively.

**106** (a) Geographic tongue (glossitis migrans).
(b) No treatment is required other than reassurance.
(c) There are no complications.

**107** (a) Accessory auricles.
(b) The 6 tubercles of His.
(c) Excision — for cosmetic reasons.

**108** (a) A pedunculated papilloma attached to the uvula.
(b) These are usually symptom-free and chance findings.

**109** (a) A pale blue, sessile, cystic swelling.
(b) This is characteristic of a ranula.
(c) Marsupialisation or more radical excision if this is extending deeply into the floor of the mouth — a 'plunging' ranula.

**110** (a) This x-ray shows occlusion of the air space of the postnasal space and oropharynx.
(b) The common cause of this appearance in a child is bulk of tonsillar and adenoid lymphoid tissue.
(c) The predominant symptom will be nasal obstruction as manifested by conspicuous snoring. Sleep apnoea may be present.

**111** (a) A left aural polyp.
(b) This protrusion of middle ear mucosa has almost certainly developed through a long-standing perforation of the tympanic membrane with an underlying chronic suppurative otitis media.
(c) Aural polypectomy, possibly followed by mastoid exploration.

**112** (a) The helix.
(b) Darwin's tubercle.
(c) No: this was described by Woolmer.

**113** (a) These are 'chalk patches' (tympanosclerosis).
(b) These may be chance findings with no apparent past history of ear disease. They are, however, invariably associated with past otitis media or previous tympanic membrane trauma or perforation. The hearing may well be normal but if extensive, these areas of tympanosclerosis may cause drum and ossicular immobility with conductive hearing loss.

**114** (a) Upper respiratory tract obstruction, particularly the common cold tends to predispose to barotrauma, particularly if there is an unawareness of descent — e.g. while asleep.
(b) The abnormal sign in this tympanic membrane is of haemorrhage along the handle of the malleus. The pressure from barotrauma has caused the rupture of a superficial vessel, leading to this small haematoma.
(c) The prognosis of simple haematoma in the absence of middle ear fluid is good — the rapid settling of the ear discomfort after the aeroplane flight and the return to a normal tympanic membrane in a matter of days.

**115** (a) Globus pharyngeus.
(b) Ask whether the symptom of discomfort in the throat is most marked when swallowing solids, liquids or saliva. A patient with globus will consistently reply that the symptom is non-existant during the swallowing of food and liquids, but is present while swallowing saliva.
(c) A barium swallow and meal is a necessary investigation. This may well confirm a cricopharyngeal spasm which is pathognomonic of globus pharyngeus. Although this problem is usually non-organic, cricopharyngeal spasm may be triggered by gastric reflux or lower oesophageal or gastric

pathology. It should not, therefore, be labelled non-organic until these sites are known to be free of significant pathology.

**116** (a) Sub-glottic stenosis. The white cicatricial ring is characteristic.
(b) Prolonged endotracheal intubation may set up subglottic inflammation and fibrosis leading to this stenosis. Direct trauma to the trachea either via direct injury or tracheostomy carried out 'too high' are the causes.

**117** (a) A barium swallow showing the pharynx and upper oesophagus.
(b) The barium is 'nipped' at the level of the cricoid — a typical example of cricopharyngeal muscle spasm (globus pharyngeus).
(c) This muscle spasm may be triggered by prominent osteophytes of the cervical spine in the region of C5/6. Pathology in the lower oesophagus or stomach, such as gastric reflux or neoplasm, may also trigger this spasm. It is, however, in most cases innocent and non-organic being perpetuated and accentuated by an over-awareness and concern about throat pathology.

**118** (a) Pneumatic otoscope.
(b) An air-filled compressible bulb is being pressed by the examiner's right hand causing air movement, to test the drum mobility,
(c) This technique is useful in diagnosing serous otitis media (glue ear). The presence of middle ear fluid reduces or renders the drum immobile. Reduced drum mobility may also be seen in the relatively rare condition of malleus fixation. A thin membrane closing a previous perforation may at first sight not be apparent and a diagnosis of a drum defect made. Air however moving the thin membrane produces a light reflex and enables the examiner to diagnose confidently that the drum is intact.

**119** (a) The columella of the nose.
(b) Reconstruction of the columella is not easy and it is rarely possible to give a result that looks completely 'non-surgical'.
(c) Composite grafts taken from the ear including cartilage and skin may be employed. Flaps, either from the nasolabial folds or from the forehead will almost certainly be required. (The loss of the columella skin in this case was self-induced during a disturbed childhood in which a habit of 'picking' the nose developed.)

**120** (a) Surgical emphysema of the soft tissues surrounding the orbit.
(b) A nasal injury in which a fracture across the ethmoid bones has linked the nasal cavity to the orbit. Air can therefore be forced from the nasal cavities into the orbital soft tissues.
(c) Crepitus.

**121** (a) The circumvallate papillae of the tongue on which the taste buds are concentrated.
(b) These papillae are supplied by the glossopharyngeal nerve.
(c) Circumvallate papillae are anterior to the sulcus terminalis and, therefore, on the anterior two-thirds of the tongue. They have, however, 'taken' the nerve supply of the posterior third of the tongue — the glossopharyngeal nerve, and are not supplied by the lingual nerve.

**122** (a) A flaring of the left alar base with some obliteration of the nasolabial groove on the left side.
(b) A cystic swelling in this site is diagnostic of a naso-alveolar cyst.
(c) Excision via a sub-labial incision.

**123** (a) A markedly retracted columella, with some flattening of the nasal tip.
(b) A septal haematoma or infected septal haematoma leads to a loss of the cartilage of the septum with columella retraction and loss of tip support.

**124** (a) Maxillary sinusitis.
(b) Frontal headache, sometimes made more severe by leaning forwards, persisting nasal obstruction, discomfort over the upper teeth on that side.
(c) Sinus x-rays and a swab of the purulent exudate for culture and sensitivity.
(d) A nasal vaso-constrictor spray (or drops), antibiotics and possibly inhalations. If there is no improvement, an antral washout is needed.

**125** (a) An unusually long and bulky uvula.
(b) This is frequently a chance finding and of no significance. It may however be associated with conspicuous snoring.
((c) Conspicuous snoring may call for sleep study investigations to exclude sleep apnoea.
(d) Uvulo-palatoplasty may be necessary if the snoring is associated with sleep apnoea. This involves excision of the uvula and shortening of the soft palate with reduction in size of the fauces.

**126** (a) Aphthous ulcer.
(b) The aetiology is unknown. Minor trauma, often dental in origin, is frequently a trigger in those susceptible to aphthous ulcers. They also tend to occur at times of tiredness or stress.
(c) There is no specific treatment for these ulcers although a corticosteroid may be used either as a lozenge or ointment.

**127** (a) The nasal bones.
(b) The upper lateral cartilage.
(c) The alar cartilage.
(d) The anterior nasal spine.

**128** (a) Stenosis of the left nasal vestibule.
(b) Chemical cautery using an agent such as trichloracetic acid. This and other similar chemical agents need to be applied precisely and with great care that they do not spread. In this case trichloracetic acid was used over a wide area of the nasal vestibule and resulted in this stenosis.
(c) The main technique for cautery in Little's area is electrocautery. Silver nitrate, chromic acid, as well as trichloracetic acid are chemicals used to deal with prominent vessels giving rise to bleeding in Little's area.

**129** (a) A haematoma of the pinna.
(b) Aspiration and a pressure dressing or excision and drainage is required.
(c) The prognosis is good, but return to a completely normal pinna may not be achieved and an early 'cauliflower ear' with some thickening of the cartilage of the pinna may result.

**130** (a) A grey opalescent swelling.
(b) This appearance is characteristic of a simple nasal polyp.
(c) A sinus x-ray may be helpful.
(d) Surgical excision and a pathological examination.

**131** (a) Familial telangiectasia.
(b) Other similar telangiectasia may be found on the body and particularly on the palms of the hands.

(c) The treatment of this condition is difficult. Cautery to the vessels may be effective and the laser may also be helpful. Removal of the septal mucosa and skin grafting is advocated. Oestrogen therapy has also been used to control severe epistaxis.

**132** (a) The lateral crus of the alar cartilage.
(b) Rhinoplasty.

**133** (a) A poorly formed or absent antihelix.
(b) Age five — or prior to starting school, when teasing, particularly amongst boys, is common.

**134** (a) Rhinoplasty.
(b) A polly-beak deformity (*Le bec du corbin* in France).
(c) Excessive removal of the nasal bone hump. Inadequate lowering of the dorsum of the septal and upper lateral cartilages.

**135** (a) The 'saddle' nose.
(b) Direct injury causing a septal haematoma: subsequent infection of this haematoma will almost certainly result in a saddle deformity; or surgical trauma in the form of a submucous resection or septoplasty in which excess septal cartilage is removed and leads to lack of support to the nasal dorsum.
(c) Sarcoid, tuberculosis, syphyllis.

**136** (a) A laryngeal tomogram.
(b) Obliteration of the normal anatomy and outline of the ventricular bands, vocal cords and subglottic narrowing.
(c) Carcinoma of the larynx. Sarcoid. Scleroma.
(d) Hoarseness. Stridor.

**137** (a) Localised dermatitis of the ear lobe.
(b) Sensitivity to an earring metal or earring sleeper.
(c) Tender cervical lymphadenopathy.

**138** (a) A preauricular sinus.
(b) A previous attempt at surgical incision.
(c) Revision operation with possible use of a skin flap for closure.

**139** (a) Absence of the fungiform papillae on the right side of the tongue, well-defined to the mid-line.
(b) The chorda tympani nerve.
(c) The chorda tympani nerve supplies taste to the anterior two-thirds of the tongue excluding the circumvallate papillae. It also carries the parasympathetic secretomotor nerve supply to the submandibular, sublingual and all the minor salivary glands in the floor of the mouth on that side.

**140** (a) The jugulodigastric or tonsillar lymph node.
(b) Acute tonsillitis with conspicuous cervical lymphadenopathy.

**141** (a) Basal cell carcinoma.
(b) Biopsy.
(c) Excision with clear margins would lead to a defect for which repair would not be straightforward in this extremely obvious site. A composite graft taken from the ear is one possibility. Radiotherapy with the linear accelerator is another possibility, as the problem of underlying cartilage necrosis is minimal with this modality.

**142** (a) This white area represents a change from nasal mucous membrane to squamous epithelium.
(b) Little's area on the anterior septum.
(c) The septal deviation to the right means that the overlying nasal mucosa is vulnerable to repeated trauma from nose-blowing and cleaning of the nose. A vestibulitis ensues and in time the nasal mucosa is replaced with squamous epithelium giving this white appearance.

**143** (a) Otitis externa (eczematous type).
(b) A swab for culture and sensitivity.
(c) This type of extensive eczema may have occurred spontaneously but may have been accentuated by the use of an antibiotic drop to which the patient is sensitive. Chloromycetin (particularly in propylene glycol) is one such cause, and neomycin topically also gives rise on occasions to this problem. This may be an isolated eczema or associated with seborrhoeic dermatitis and eczema elsewhere.

**144** (a) Torus palatinus.
(b) Characteristically mid-line, bony-hard on the hard palate, and rather hot-cross-bun in shape.
(c) No treatment is required unless the swelling is of sufficient size to cause symptoms through its bulk or interfere with the fitting of a denture.

**145** (a) The margin of the lateral crus of the alar cartilage.
(b) Nasal tip deformity. The rhinoplasty operation modifies or alters the anatomy of this structure in various tip deformities.

**146** (a) The cartilage of the cavum concha of the ear.
(b) This elastic cartilage is extremely useful in nasal reconstruction when there has been loss of nasal cartilage.

**147** (a) Alar collapse on inspiration due to a narrow or 'weak' side wall of the nasal vestibule.
(b) This is quite common bilaterally when the nares are narrow and the side wall of the nose is flaccid. It may follow rhinoplasty surgery in which an excess of lateral crus of the alar cartilage has been removed. It is, however, very unusual to see this occurring on one side only as demonstrated here.
(c) A composite cartilage graft taken from the cavum concha of the ear is one technique for supporting the side wall of the nose in this type of nasal obstruction.

**148** (a) Deviation of the nasal bones to the left. A subconjunctival haemorrhage in the left eye with periorbital haematoma (palpation and x-rays should be carried out to exclude an associated fracture in the region of the orbit).
(b) A septal haematoma (a septal deviation will not cause total obstruction on both sides).
(c) Watery rhinorrhoea should arouse the suspicion of a CSF leak. Purulent rhinorrhoea suggests a sinusitis related to infected haematoma in one of the sinuses.

**149** (a) Widening of the nasal bones.
(b) Nasal polypi, if extensive, will cause expansion of the nasal bones and give rise to this characteristic widening.

**150** (a) A red swelling at the orifice of the submandibular duct (Wharton's duct).
(b) An impacted calculus at the orifice of Wharton's duct.
(c) Incision overlying the calculus with enucleation.


**151** (a) Glue ear or chronic secretory otitis media.
(b) Audiometry post-operatively shows normal hearing provided the grommet is patent, free of infection without discharge, and in satisfactory position.
(c) Over nine months.
(d) Insertion of grommets is the commonest operation in the world at present.


**152** (a) It is better for the patient to be sat up and leaning forwards. A patient lying down with epistaxis tends to swallow the blood which leads to epigastric pain, nausea and possible vomiting.
(b) Pressure over the side wall of the nose sustained for 3-4 minutes.
(c) Most epistaxis is from Little's area (or Kiesselbach's plexus).
(d) Vessels from the superior labial artery, anterior ethmoidal artery, spheno-palatine artery and greater palatine artery supply this area of the nose.


**153** (a) Collapse of the lateral crus of the alar cartilage causing narrowing of the nasal vestibule. This is a so-called 'pinched' nose.
(b) The patient will complain of nasal obstruction on inspiration.
(c) Excessive removal of the lateral crus of the alar cartilage (probably associated with overlying vestibular skin) may have been attempted during a rhinoplasty operation and carried out to excess to narrow the nasal tip.
(d) Surgery with the use of a composite graft to enlarge the nasal vestibule, or an indwelling nasal dilator.


**154** (a) The fact that this granulation tissue is mid-line and sub-mental are the key characteristics for spot diagnosis.
(b) Examination of the lower incisor teeth for obvious caries or tenderness on percussion. An x-ray to show the apices of the lower incisor teeth.
(c) An apical abscess involving the lower incisor tooth with a sinus tracking through the sub-mental region where granulation tissue lies at the opening of this sinus.


**155** (a) A dull red swelling occupies the anterior hypotympanum.
(b) Pulsation and blanching if the pneumatic otoscope is used.
(c) This appearance of a pulsating swelling in the hypotympanum is characteristic of a glomus jugulare tumour (a chemodectoma) or paraganglioma.


**156** (a) A lateral soft tissue x-ray of the neck.
(b) A very gross swelling of the pre-cervical soft tissue area (or retropharyngeal space). Air is apparent.
(c) A perforation of the upper oesophagus either with a foreign body (such as a fish or meat bone) or following oesophagoscopy.

**157** (a) This barium swallow demonstrates a moderate sized pharyngeal pouch or diverticulum.

(b) Dysphagia with a pouch may vary from no symptoms to absolute dysphagia (when the pouch becomes impacted with food and debris pressing on the upper oesophagus). Some gurgling or noisy swallowing may be associated with a pouch but this would probably not be sufficiently large to produce swelling in the neck.

(c) A cough is commonly associated with a pouch from overspill, particularly when lying down at night. Overspill may also give rise to either a pulmonary abscess or pulmonary fibrosis (giving a chest x-ray picture similar to tuberculosis from multiple small areas of pulmonary fibrosis following infection from small 'spills').

**158** (a) Yellow cystic swellings are apparent on both tonsils near the superior poles. These are typical retention cysts.

(b) These are usually symptom-free and chance findings. Concern by the patient when they have noticed this lesion is usually the cause of referral.

(c) Treatment is normally unnecessary, other than reassurance, but if these cysts increase in size and give symptoms from their bulk, or extreme concern to the patient, tonsillectomy or 'de-roofing' the cysts is necessary.

**159** (a) This x-ray demonstrates three calculi in the submandibular duct (Wharton's duct).

(b) Symptoms associated with submandibular calculi are usually intermittent swelling of the submandibular gland, at times of salvation, associated with discomfort or pain.

(c) Calculi in the duct can usually be removed via an intraoral incision over Wharton's duct. Suturing of this incision is not necessary and may, in fact, lead to duct stenosis.

**160** (a) A submandibular sialogram.

(b) Submandibular sialography is relatively rarely used or necessary. This procedure is not easy to carry out as the submandibular duct is considerably more difficult to cannulate than the parotid duct. The orifice is small and elusive for cannulation compared to the parotid duct.

(c) This sialogram demonstrates sialectasia — more common in the parotid gland. Dilated ducts give an appearance similar to bronchiectasis and intermittent painful swelling of the submandibular gland is characteristic of this condition, for which excision of the gland may be necessary.

**161** (a) A submandibular calculus impacted as the submandibular duct exits from the gland, is apparent.

(b) Intermittent or permanent tender swelling of the submandibular gland, more marked at times of salivation, would be the presenting symptom.

(c) Excision of the submandibular gland is necessary in this case, as the stone is within the substance of the gland and not accessible via an intraoral incision over the submandibular duct in the floor of the mouth.

**162** The lateral swelling is a conspicuous anterior end of the inferior turbinate. The more medial swelling is grey and opalescent and characteristic of a simple 'allergic-type' nasal polyp.

**163** (a) A swelling is apparent in the upper third of the neck, partly concealed by the fibres of the sternomastoid muscle.

(b) The site of this swelling is characteristic of a branchial cyst.

(c) Excision.
(d) The internal jugular vein is closely related to the deep surface of the branchial cyst and dissection of this lesion from the vein will be necessary.

**164** (a) This x-ray shows a foreign body in the region of the cricopharyngeal sphincter of the upper oesophagus — one of the commonest sites for the impaction of foreign bodies such as a bone as in this instance.
(b) Removal by oesophagoscopy is necessary.
(c) An oesophageal perforation. Pain, which may be referred to the ear or the mid-line of the neck posteriorly. Dysphagia, fever and possible neck emphysema with stiffness of the neck may be associated with a foreign body.

**165** (a) Xanthelasma.
(b) Serum lipids.
(c) Excision with undermining and closure. Skin grafting if the area is too large for primary closure may be necessary.
(d) Ectropion.

**166** (a) The right tonsil is conspicuously larger than the left. It does not appear to have been 'pushed' medially by a para-phalangeal swelling.
(b) The severe sore throat may well have been a quinsy and the persistent discomfort may be due to a chronic quinsy. With unilateral tonsilar enlargement however, the question of a neoplasm must not be overlooked.
(c) Tonsillectomy/biopsy would be the treatment necessary.

**167** (a) A mixed parotid tumour (pleomorphic adenoma).
(b) It is necessary to check the facial nerve movement (VIIth cranial nerve). A more highly malignant parotid gland tumour will involve the facial nerve, causing some facial weakness.
(c) Superficial parotidectomy with preservation of the facial nerve is the treatment for a parotid pleomorphic adenoma.

**168** (a) An associated septal deviation is almost certainly present with such a gross external nasal deformity. Nasal obstruction is therefore certain to be either the presenting symptom or the symptom associated with a dislike of the external deformity of the nose.
(b) A rhinoplasty and septoplasty may well be necessary.

**169** (a) Rodent cell carcinoma (basal cell carcinoma).
(b) Radiotherapy, surgical excision or Moh's excision.
(c) The prognosis is excellent. A small non-adherent basal cell carcinoma is normally curable.

**170** (a) This lesion followed discharge and discomfort after earring piercing.
(b) The histology showed infected granulation tissue.

**171** (a) There is an obvious severe deviation/dislocation of the caudal end of the cartilagenous septum into the right nasal vestibule with a more posterior deviation into the left nasal fossa.
(b) A past history of trauma to the nose is probable with such a severe and obvious dislocation and there may be an associated external deviation of the nose.
(c) Septal surgery — a septoplasty.

**172** (a) There is a vestibulitis with an eczematous reaction of the skin of the tip of the nose.

(b) A granular-type rhinitis may be associated with this finding in which the nasal mucosa is hyperaemic and uneven in appearance.

(c) This type of nasal vestibulitis and granular rhinitis may be associated with autoimmune diseases such as disseminated lupus erythematosis, polyarteritis nodosa or AIDS.

**173** (a) The submandibular duct (Wharton's duct) and the lingual nerve, which loops around it, are the arrowed structures.

(b) The nerve, superficial to the submandibular gland, at risk during excision is the mandibular branch of the facial nerve.

(c) The bottom lip on the side of the injury does not lower when the mouth is opened. Asymmetry of the lip movement on smiling and talking is noticeable if the mandibular branch of the facial nerve is damaged.

**174** (a) In a child a clear view of the anterior nares is often obtained with simple pressure on the nasal tip with the thumb — rather than using a nasal speculum. In this instance a gross dislocation of the caudal end of the septal cartilage is apparent with an overlying vestibulitis of the vestibular skin.

(b) Crusting, 'soreness' with occasional epistaxis associated with nasal obstruction on that side, are the symptoms to be anticipated.

(c) Septal surgery in children is best avoided unless the nasal obstruction is gross, in which case a limited septoplasty is carried out to improve the airway. Antibiotic/corticosteroid ointment may well be helpful for the vestibulitis, along with advice to avoid unnecessary trauma on cleaning or blowing the nose, so that this skin is not unnecessarily excoriated.

**175** (a) A right facial palsy (lower motor neurone, as the entire face is involved including the forehead) is apparent.

(b) A Bell's palsy is the commonest type of facial palsy.

(c) Some transient sharp pain in the right ear may precede Bell's palsy, and alteration in taste due to involvement of the chorda tympani may precede or be associated with Bell's palsy.

(d) Prognosis for most Bell's palsies is good. Corticosteroid treatment in the early stages probably improves the prognosis.

# Index

Numbers refer not to pages, but to the number shared by the illustration, question and answer.